MIND DIET COOKBOOK

FOR SENIORS OVER 60

1000 Days Of Flavorful Recipes for a Sharp and Vibrant Mind

Mara Tromp

COPYRIGHT

Table of Contents

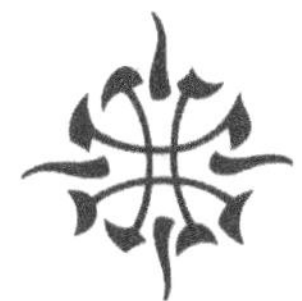

Chapter 1

Introduction to the MIND Diet for Seniors

BENEFITS OF THE MIND DIET FOR COGNITIVE HEALTH IN SENIORS

The MIND diet, which stands for Mediterranean-DASH Diet Intervention for Neurodegenerative Delay, is a dietary pattern specifically designed to promote brain health and reduce the risk of cognitive decline, particularly in seniors. It combines elements of the Mediterranean diet and the DASH (Dietary Approaches to Stop Hypertension) diet, both of which have been independently associated with numerous health benefits. By incorporating key nutrients and food groups that are believed to support brain function, the MIND diet offers several potential benefits for cognitive health in seniors.

1. Reduced risk of cognitive decline: The MIND diet emphasizes foods that have been shown to be beneficial for brain health. This diet encourages the consumption of leafy green vegetables, berries, whole grains, nuts, beans, olive oil, fish, and poultry, while limiting the intake of red meat, butter and margarine, cheese, pastries, sweets, and fried and fast food. Many of these recommended foods are rich in antioxidants, anti-inflammatory compounds, and essential nutrients, which have been associated with a lower risk of cognitive decline and neurodegenerative diseases like Alzheimer's.

2. Protection against oxidative stress: Oxidative stress, which occurs when there is an imbalance between the production of free radicals and the body's ability to neutralize them, is thought to play a role in age-related cognitive decline. The MIND diet includes foods that are high in antioxidants, such as berries, leafy greens, and nuts. Antioxidants help combat oxidative stress by neutralizing free radicals and reducing inflammation, potentially protecting brain cells from damage and supporting cognitive function.

3. Improved cardiovascular health: The MIND diet incorporates elements of the Mediterranean and DASH diets, both of which have been associated with improved cardiovascular health. By emphasizing the consumption of fruits, vegetables, whole grains, and healthy fats like olive oil, while limiting saturated and trans fats, the MIND diet can

help seniors maintain healthy blood pressure levels, reduce cholesterol levels, and lower the risk of heart disease and stroke. Improved cardiovascular health is closely linked to better cognitive function, as a healthy blood supply is crucial for delivering oxygen and nutrients to the brain.

4. Enhanced nutrient intake: The MIND diet encourages the consumption of nutrient-dense foods, providing seniors with a wide range of essential vitamins, minerals, and phytochemicals. For example, leafy greens like spinach and kale are rich in folate, vitamin K, and antioxidants, which are believed to support cognitive function. Berries, particularly blueberries, are packed with flavonoids and other compounds that have been shown to improve memory and learning. Omega-3 fatty acids found in fish like salmon and tuna are important for brain health and have been associated with a reduced risk of cognitive decline.

5. Long-term sustainability: One of the advantages of the MIND diet is its focus on incorporating healthy eating patterns that are sustainable in the long term. Unlike restrictive diets, the MIND diet allows for flexibility and includes a variety of delicious and nutrient-rich foods. This makes it more feasible for seniors to adopt and adhere to the diet, which is crucial for reaping its cognitive health benefits over time.

6. Positive impact on overall health: The MIND diet not only supports cognitive health but also promotes overall well-being. By encouraging the consumption of whole, unprocessed foods and discouraging the intake of unhealthy fats and processed snacks, the MIND diet can help seniors maintain a healthy weight, manage chronic conditions like diabetes and hypertension, and reduce the risk of other age-related ailments, such as certain types of cancer and neurodegenerative diseases.

In conclusion, the MIND diet offers numerous potential benefits for cognitive health in seniors. By emphasizing nutrient-dense foods and incorporating elements of the Mediterranean and DASH diets, it provides a balanced and sustainable approach to promoting brain health and reducing the risk of cognitive decline. However, it is important to note that while the MIND diet shows promise, individual results may vary, and it should be complemented with other lifestyle factors such as regular physical exercise, mental stimulation, and social engagement to maximize its effectiveness in maintaining cognitive function in seniors.

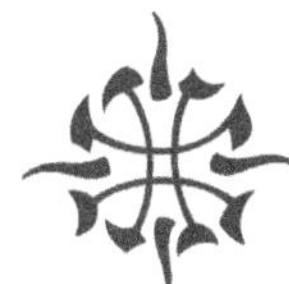

Chapter 2

Breakfast Recipes

BLUEBERRY OATMEAL BREAKFAST BOWL

Blueberry Oatmeal Breakfast Bowl is a nutritious and delicious way to start your day. Packed with fiber, antioxidants, and essential nutrients, this recipe combines the goodness of oats and blueberries to provide a fulfilling and energizing breakfast. Here's a simple recipe to help you make a delightful Blueberry Oatmeal Breakfast Bowl:

Ingredients:

- 1/2 cup rolled oats

- 1 cup water or milk of your choice (e.g., dairy milk, almond milk, soy milk)

- 1/2 cup fresh or frozen blueberries

- 1 tablespoon honey or maple syrup (optional)

- A pinch of salt

- Toppings of your choice, such as sliced almonds, chia seeds, flaxseeds, or shredded coconut

Instructions:

1. In a saucepan, bring the water or milk to a boil over medium heat.

2. Add the rolled oats and a pinch of salt to the boiling liquid. Stir well.

3. Reduce the heat to low and let the oats simmer for about 5 minutes, stirring occasionally. If you prefer a thicker consistency, cook for a few more minutes.

4. Once the oats have cooked to your desired consistency, remove the saucepan from heat.

5. Stir in the honey or maple syrup (if using) to sweeten the oatmeal.

6. Gently fold in the blueberries, reserving a few for garnish.

7. Transfer the oatmeal to a serving bowl.

8. Sprinkle your choice of toppings over the oatmeal. Sliced almonds, chia seeds, flaxseeds, or shredded coconut work well.

9. Finally, garnish with the reserved blueberries.

Your Blueberry Oatmeal Breakfast Bowl is now ready to be enjoyed! Feel free to customize the recipe by adding additional toppings like sliced bananas, a dollop of yogurt, or a sprinkle of cinnamon for extra flavor. This recipe can be easily doubled or adjusted to suit your preferences. It's a wholesome and satisfying breakfast that will keep you fueled and focused throughout the morning.

Remember, breakfast is an important meal, so starting your day with a nutrient-packed bowl like this can contribute to your overall well-being and provide you with the energy you need to tackle the day ahead.

Sure! Here are two additional breakfast recipes: Spinach and Feta Omelette and Whole Grain Banana Walnut Pancakes.

SPINACH AND FETA OMELETTE

Ingredients

- 3 large eggs

- 1/4 cup crumbled feta cheese

- 1 cup fresh spinach leaves

- 1/4 cup diced tomatoes

- 1/4 cup diced red bell pepper

- 1 tablespoon chopped fresh herbs (such as basil, parsley, or chives)

- Salt and pepper to taste

- 1 tablespoon olive oil or cooking spray

Instructions

1. In a bowl, whisk the eggs until well beaten. Season with salt and pepper to taste.

2. Heat the olive oil or cooking spray in a non-stick skillet over medium heat.

3. Add the diced red bell pepper to the skillet and sauté for 2-3 minutes until slightly softened.

4. Add the fresh spinach leaves to the skillet and cook until wilted, about 2 minutes.

5. Pour the beaten eggs over the vegetables in the skillet, ensuring that they are evenly distributed.

6. Sprinkle the crumbled feta cheese, diced tomatoes, and chopped fresh herbs over the eggs.

7. Cook the omelette for 3-4 minutes or until the bottom is set and the edges are slightly browned.

8. Carefully flip half of the omelette over the other half using a spatula.

9. Cook for another 2-3 minutes until the omelette is fully cooked and the cheese has melted.

10. Slide the omelette onto a plate and fold it in half. Serve hot and enjoy a nutritious and flavorful Spinach and Feta Omelette!

Whole Grain Banana Walnut Pancakes

Ingredients

- 1 cup whole wheat flour

- 1 tablespoon ground flaxseed (optional)

- 1 teaspoon baking powder

- 1/2 teaspoon baking soda

- 1/4 teaspoon salt

- 1 ripe banana, mashed

- 1 cup buttermilk (or substitute with milk of your choice)

- 1 large egg

- 1 tablespoon honey or maple syrup

- 1/2 teaspoon vanilla extract

- 1/4 cup chopped walnuts

- Cooking spray or butter for greasing the pan

Instructions

1. In a large bowl, whisk together the whole wheat flour, ground flaxseed (if using), baking powder, baking soda, and salt.

2. In a separate bowl, mash the ripe banana until smooth. Add the buttermilk, egg, honey or maple syrup, and vanilla extract. Whisk until well combined.

3. Pour the wet ingredients into the dry ingredients and stir until just combined. Be careful not to overmix; a few lumps are okay. Fold in the chopped walnuts.

4. Heat a non-stick skillet or griddle over medium heat and lightly coat it with cooking spray or butter.

5. Pour 1/4 cup of batter onto the skillet for each pancake. Cook until bubbles form on the surface, then flip and cook for an additional 1-2 minutes until golden brown.

6. Repeat the process with the remaining batter, greasing the skillet as needed.

7. Serve the pancakes warm with additional sliced bananas, a drizzle of honey or maple syrup, and a sprinkle of chopped walnuts on top.

These Whole Grain Banana Walnut Pancakes are a wholesome and tasty way to start your day, providing a good balance of whole grains, fruit, and healthy fats. Enjoy them as a delightful breakfast treat!

Avocado Toast with Smoked Salmon

Ingredients:

- 2 slices of whole grain bread

- 1 ripe avocado

- Juice of 1/2 lemon

- Salt and pepper to taste

- 2 ounces smoked salmon

- 1 tablespoon chopped fresh dill (optional)

- Red pepper flakes (optional)

Instructions

1. Toast the slices of whole grain bread to your desired level of crispness.

2. While the bread is toasting, cut the ripe avocado in half lengthwise. Remove the pit and scoop the flesh into a bowl.

3. Add the lemon juice, salt, and pepper to the avocado. Mash the avocado with a fork until you achieve your desired consistency. Some prefer a smooth texture, while others prefer a chunkier avocado mixture.

4. Once the bread is toasted, spread the mashed avocado evenly on each slice.

5. Place the smoked salmon on top of the avocado layer, dividing it evenly between the two slices.

6. Sprinkle the chopped fresh dill and red pepper flakes (if desired) over the smoked salmon.

7. Serve the Avocado Toast with Smoked Salmon immediately and enjoy the combination of creamy avocado, smoky salmon, and fresh flavors!

Greek Yogurt Parfait with Berries and Almonds

Ingredients:

- 1 cup Greek yogurt

- 1 tablespoon honey or maple syrup

- 1/2 teaspoon vanilla extract

- 1 cup mixed berries (such as strawberries, blueberries, and raspberries)

- 1/4 cup sliced almonds

- 2 tablespoons granola (optional)

Instructions:

1. In a bowl, combine the Greek yogurt, honey or maple syrup, and vanilla extract. Stir well to incorporate the sweetener and vanilla into the yogurt.

2. Wash and prepare the mixed berries by rinsing them under cold water and removing any stems or leaves. If the berries are large, you can slice them into smaller pieces.

3. In a glass or bowl, layer the Greek yogurt mixture, mixed berries, sliced almonds, and granola (if using). Start with a layer of yogurt, followed by a layer of berries, then a sprinkle of almonds, and repeat until the ingredients are used.

4. Finish the parfait with a dollop of Greek yogurt and a few extra berries on top for an attractive presentation.

5. Serve the Greek Yogurt Parfait with Berries and Almonds immediately, or refrigerate for a few hours to allow the flavors to meld together.

This delightful parfait offers a balance of creamy yogurt, juicy berries, crunchy almonds, and a touch of sweetness. It's a nutritious and satisfying breakfast option that will keep you energized throughout the morning. Enjoy!

VEGGIE BREAKFAST BURRITO

Ingredients

- 1 large tortilla wrap (whole wheat or flour)

- 2 large eggs

- 1/4 cup diced bell peppers (red, green, or a mix)

- 1/4 cup diced onions

- 1/4 cup sliced mushrooms

- 1/4 cup diced tomatoes

- 1/4 cup shredded cheddar cheese

- 1 tablespoon olive oil

- Salt and pepper to taste

- Optional toppings: salsa, avocado slices, sour cream

Instructions

1. Heat the olive oil in a skillet over medium heat. Add the diced onions and bell peppers and sauté until they are slightly softened, about 3-4 minutes.

2. Add the sliced mushrooms to the skillet and cook for an additional 2-3 minutes until they are tender.

3. In a bowl, beat the eggs and season with salt and pepper.

4. Push the sautéed vegetables to one side of the skillet and pour the beaten eggs onto the other side.

5. Scramble the eggs, stirring occasionally until they are fully cooked and no longer runny.

6. Warm the tortilla in a separate pan or microwave for a few seconds to make it pliable.

7. Place the scrambled eggs on the tortilla, followed by the diced tomatoes and shredded cheese.

8. If desired, add optional toppings such as salsa, avocado slices, or sour cream.

9. Fold the sides of the tortilla inward and roll it up tightly to form a burrito shape.

10. Cut the Veggie Breakfast Burrito in half diagonally and serve it warm. Enjoy a delicious and satisfying breakfast on the go!

Quinoa Breakfast Porridge with Mixed Berries

Ingredients

- 1/2 cup quinoa

- 1 cup water

- 1 cup milk of your choice (e.g., dairy milk, almond milk, soy milk)

- 1 tablespoon honey or maple syrup

- 1/2 teaspoon vanilla extract

- 1 cup mixed berries (such as strawberries, blueberries, and raspberries)

- 2 tablespoons chopped nuts (e.g., almonds, walnuts, or pecans)

- Optional toppings: a sprinkle of cinnamon, a drizzle of honey

Instructions:

1. Rinse the quinoa under cold water to remove any bitterness.

2. In a saucepan, combine the rinsed quinoa and water. Bring to a boil over medium heat.

3. Reduce the heat to low, cover the saucepan, and simmer for 15-20 minutes or until the quinoa is tender and the liquid is absorbed.

4. Once the quinoa is cooked, stir in the milk, honey or maple syrup, and vanilla extract. Cook for an additional 3-4 minutes until the mixture is heated through.

5. Divide the Quinoa Breakfast Porridge among serving bowls.

6. Top each bowl with a generous amount of mixed berries and sprinkle with chopped nuts.

7. If desired, add optional toppings such as a sprinkle of cinnamon or a drizzle of honey for extra flavor.

8. Serve the Quinoa Breakfast Porridge with Mixed Berries warm and enjoy a wholesome breakfast packed with protein, fiber, and antioxidants!

These breakfast recipes offer a variety of flavors and nutrients to start your day off right. Whether you prefer a savory burrito or a sweet and nourishing porridge, these recipes will provide you with a delicious and satisfying breakfast experience. Enjoy!

Certainly! Here are two more breakfast recipes: Almond Butter and Banana Smoothie and Chia Seed Pudding with Mango and Coconut.

ALMOND BUTTER AND BANANA SMOOTHIE

Ingredients:

- 1 ripe banana

- 2 tablespoons almond butter

- 1 cup almond milk (or milk of your choice)

- 1 tablespoon honey or maple syrup (optional, for added sweetness)

- 1/2 teaspoon vanilla extract

- 1/2 cup ice cubes

Instructions

1. Peel the ripe banana and break it into chunks.

2. In a blender, combine the banana chunks, almond butter, almond milk, honey or maple syrup (if using), vanilla extract, and ice cubes.

3. Blend on high speed until all the ingredients are well combined and the smoothie is creamy and smooth.

4. Taste the smoothie and adjust the sweetness by adding more honey or maple syrup if desired.

5. Pour the Almond Butter and Banana Smoothie into a glass and serve it immediately. It's a delicious and nutritious way to start your day!

CHIA SEED PUDDING WITH MANGO AND COCONUT

Ingredients

- 1/4 cup chia seeds

- 1 cup coconut milk (or milk of your choice)

- 1 tablespoon honey or maple syrup

- 1/2 teaspoon vanilla extract

- 1 ripe mango, diced

- 2 tablespoons shredded coconut

Instructions:

1. In a bowl, combine the chia seeds, coconut milk, honey or maple syrup, and vanilla extract. Stir well to evenly distribute the chia seeds.

2. Let the mixture sit for 5 minutes, then stir again to prevent clumping. Repeat this process once or twice more over the next 15 minutes.

3. Cover the bowl and refrigerate for at least 2 hours or overnight to allow the chia seeds to absorb the liquid and create a pudding-like texture.

4. When ready to serve, give the chia seed pudding a good stir to make sure it's well mixed.

5. Divide the chia seed pudding into serving bowls or jars.

6. Top each serving with the diced mango and a sprinkle of shredded coconut.

7. Serve the Chia Seed Pudding with Mango and Coconut chilled and enjoy the refreshing combination of flavors and textures!

Both of these recipes offer a delightful and nutritious breakfast experience. The Almond Butter and Banana Smoothie provides a creamy and satisfying blend of flavors, while the Chia Seed Pudding with Mango and Coconut offers a refreshing and tropical treat. Enjoy these breakfast options to kick-start your day on a healthy note!

EGG MUFFINS WITH SPINACH AND SUN-DRIED TOMATOES

Ingredients:

- 6 large eggs

- 1/4 cup milk

- 1 cup fresh spinach, chopped

- 1/4 cup sun-dried tomatoes, chopped

- 1/4 cup shredded cheese (such as cheddar or feta)

- 1/4 teaspoon salt

- 1/4 teaspoon black pepper

- Cooking spray or butter for greasing the muffin tin

Instructions:

1. Preheat your oven to 350°F (175°C). Grease a muffin tin with cooking spray or butter to prevent sticking.

2. In a mixing bowl, crack the eggs and whisk them together until well beaten.

3. Add the milk, salt, and black pepper to the eggs and whisk until fully combined.

4. Stir in the chopped spinach, sun-dried tomatoes, and shredded cheese into the egg mixture. Make sure all the ingredients are evenly distributed.

5. Pour the egg mixture into each muffin cup, filling them about 3/4 full. Leave a little room for the egg muffins to rise while baking.

6. Place the muffin tin in the preheated oven and bake for approximately 20-25 minutes, or until the egg muffins are set and slightly golden on top. You can test doneness by inserting a toothpick into the center of one muffin—it should come out clean.

7. Once the egg muffins are done, remove the muffin tin from the oven and let them cool for a few minutes.

8. Run a knife around the edges of the muffin cups to loosen the egg muffins. Carefully remove them from the muffin tin and transfer them to a wire rack to cool completely.

9. Once cooled, the Egg Muffins with Spinach and Sun-Dried Tomatoes can be stored in an airtight container in the refrigerator for up to 3-4 days.

10. These egg muffins can be enjoyed either cold or reheated. To reheat, simply place them in a microwave-safe dish and heat on medium power for about 30 seconds to 1 minute, until warmed through.

11. Serve the Egg Muffins with Spinach and Sun-Dried Tomatoes as a delicious and protein-packed breakfast or snack option. They are convenient, portable, and customizable—feel free to add other ingredients like diced bell peppers, onions, or cooked bacon to suit your taste preferences.

Egg Muffins with Spinach and Sun-Dried Tomatoes are a versatile and nutritious option for busy mornings or as a make-ahead breakfast. Enjoy the combination of savory flavors and the boost of protein these muffins provide to start your day off right!

Chapter 3

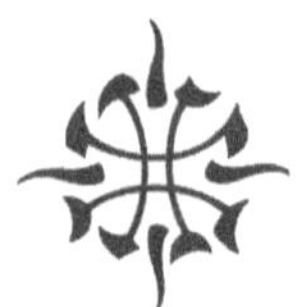

Lunch Ideas

MEDITERRANEAN CHICKPEA SALAD

Here's a recipe for Mediterranean Chickpea Salad, perfect for a healthy and refreshing lunch:

Ingredients:

- 2 cups cooked chickpeas (or 1 can, drained and rinsed)

- 1 cup cherry tomatoes, halved

- 1 cucumber, diced

- 1/2 red onion, thinly sliced

- 1/2 cup Kalamata olives, pitted and halved

- 1/4 cup crumbled feta cheese

- 1/4 cup chopped fresh parsley

- 2 tablespoons extra-virgin olive oil

- 2 tablespoons lemon juice

- 1 garlic clove, minced

- 1/2 teaspoon dried oregano

- Salt and pepper to taste

Instructions:

1. In a large mixing bowl, combine the cooked chickpeas, cherry tomatoes, cucumber, red onion, Kalamata olives, crumbled feta cheese, and chopped parsley.

2. In a small bowl, whisk together the extra-virgin olive oil, lemon juice, minced garlic, dried oregano, salt, and pepper to make the dressing.

3. Pour the dressing over the salad ingredients in the large mixing bowl.

4. Gently toss all the ingredients together until they are well coated in the dressing.

5. Taste the salad and adjust the seasoning with additional salt and pepper if needed.

6. Allow the Mediterranean Chickpea Salad to sit for at least 15-20 minutes before serving, to allow the flavors to meld together.

7. Serve the salad as a light and satisfying lunch on its own, or as a side dish alongside grilled chicken or fish.

8. If desired, you can also add additional ingredients like diced bell peppers, chopped fresh mint, or a sprinkle of dried chili flakes to customize the salad to your liking.

Mediterranean Chickpea Salad is packed with protein, fiber, and vibrant flavors. It's a nutritious and delicious option for a refreshing lunch that will keep you satisfied throughout the day. Enjoy!

SALMON NICOISE SALAD

Here's a recipe for a flavorful and nutritious Salmon Niçoise Salad:

Ingredients:

- 1 pound salmon fillets

- Salt and black pepper, to taste

- 2 tablespoons olive oil, divided

- 4 cups mixed salad greens

- 1 cup cherry tomatoes, halved

- 1 cup cooked green beans, trimmed and halved

- 1/2 cup Kalamata olives, pitted

- 4 hard-boiled eggs, peeled and halved

- 1/4 cup red onion, thinly sliced

- 2 tablespoons capers

- For the dressing:

  - 3 tablespoons lemon juice

  - 2 tablespoons Dijon mustard

  - 1 garlic clove, minced

  - 1/4 cup extra-virgin olive oil

  - Salt and black pepper, to taste

Instructions:

1. Preheat the oven to 400°F (200°C). Season the salmon fillets with salt and black pepper.

2. Heat 1 tablespoon of olive oil in an oven-safe skillet over medium-high heat. Place the salmon fillets in the skillet, skin-side down, and cook for 2-3 minutes until the skin is crispy.

3. Transfer the skillet to the preheated oven and bake for 10-12 minutes, or until the salmon is cooked through and flakes easily with a fork.

4. While the salmon is cooking, prepare the dressing. In a small bowl, whisk together the lemon juice, Dijon mustard, minced garlic, extra-virgin olive oil, salt, and black pepper until well combined.

5. In a large salad bowl, combine the mixed salad greens, cherry tomatoes, cooked green beans, Kalamata olives, hard-boiled eggs, red onion, and capers.

6. Drizzle the dressing over the salad ingredients and toss gently to coat everything evenly.

7. Once the salmon is ready, remove it from the oven and let it cool for a few minutes. Break the salmon into large flakes using a fork.

8. Add the flaked salmon to the salad bowl and gently toss to incorporate it with the other ingredients.

9. Divide the Salmon Niçoise Salad among serving plates or bowls.

10. Serve the salad immediately as a satisfying and complete lunch or dinner option.

The Salmon Niçoise Salad is a delightful combination of flavors and textures, with the richness of the salmon complemented by the freshness of the salad ingredients. It's a perfect choice for a healthy and flavorful meal. Enjoy!

Turkey and Avocado Wrap with Whole Wheat Tortilla

Here's a recipe for a delicious and nutritious Turkey and Avocado Wrap with Whole Wheat Tortilla:

Ingredients:

- 1 large whole wheat tortilla

- 4-6 slices of turkey breast

- 1/2 avocado, sliced

- 1/4 cup sliced cucumber

- 1/4 cup shredded lettuce

- 2 tablespoons mayonnaise or Greek yogurt

- 1 teaspoon Dijon mustard

- Salt and pepper, to taste

Instructions:

1. Lay the whole wheat tortilla flat on a clean surface or plate.

2. In a small bowl, mix together the mayonnaise or Greek yogurt and Dijon mustard. Season with salt and pepper to taste.

3. Spread the mayonnaise or Greek yogurt mixture evenly over the whole wheat tortilla.

4. Arrange the turkey slices on top of the tortilla, covering the surface in an even layer.

5. Place the sliced avocado, sliced cucumber, and shredded lettuce on top of the turkey slices.

6. Starting from one end, tightly roll the tortilla into a wrap, making sure the filling is secure.

7. Cut the wrap in half crosswise or into smaller pinwheels, if desired, for easier handling.

8. Serve the Turkey and Avocado Wrap immediately or wrap it tightly in foil or plastic wrap for later consumption.

9. This wrap makes a delicious and portable lunch option. You can also pack it with some fresh fruit or a side salad for a complete meal.

The Turkey and Avocado Wrap with Whole Wheat Tortilla is a balanced and satisfying choice, combining lean protein from the turkey, healthy fats from the avocado, and fiber from the whole wheat tortilla. Enjoy this tasty and nutritious wrap for a quick and easy lunch!

Certainly! Here are two lengthy recipes for Quinoa and Vegetable Stuffed Bell Peppers and Lentil Soup with Kale and Carrots:

QUINOA AND VEGETABLE STUFFED BELL PEPPERS

Ingredients

- 4 large bell peppers (any color)

- 1 cup quinoa, rinsed

- 1 3/4 cups vegetable broth or water

- 1 tablespoon olive oil

- 1 onion, diced

- 2 cloves garlic, minced

- 1 zucchini, diced

- 1 yellow squash, diced

- 1 carrot, diced

- 1 cup diced tomatoes

- 1 teaspoon dried oregano

- 1 teaspoon dried basil

- 1/2 teaspoon paprika

- Salt and pepper, to taste

- 1/2 cup shredded mozzarella cheese (optional)

- Fresh parsley, chopped (for garnish)

Instructions

1. Preheat your oven to 375°F (190°C). Prepare a baking dish by lightly greasing it with olive oil or cooking spray.

2. Cut off the tops of the bell peppers and remove the seeds and membranes. Place the bell peppers in the prepared baking dish, standing upright. Set aside.

3. In a saucepan, combine the rinsed quinoa and vegetable broth or water. Bring to a boil, then reduce the heat to low. Cover and simmer for about 15 minutes, or until the quinoa is cooked and the liquid is absorbed.

4. In a separate skillet, heat the olive oil over medium heat. Add the diced onion and minced garlic, and sauté until the onion becomes translucent and fragrant.

5. Add the diced zucchini, yellow squash, and carrot to the skillet. Cook for about 5 minutes, or until the vegetables are slightly tender.

6. Stir in the diced tomatoes, dried oregano, dried basil, paprika, salt, and pepper. Continue cooking for another 2-3 minutes to allow the flavors to meld together.

7. Remove the skillet from the heat and add the cooked quinoa to the vegetable mixture. Stir well to combine all the ingredients.

8. Spoon the quinoa and vegetable mixture into the prepared bell peppers, filling them to the top. Press down gently to pack the filling.

9. If desired, sprinkle shredded mozzarella cheese on top of each stuffed bell pepper.

10. Cover the baking dish with foil and bake for 25-30 minutes, or until the bell peppers are tender and the filling is heated through.

11. Remove the foil and continue baking for an additional 5 minutes to allow the cheese to melt and slightly brown.

12. Once done, remove the stuffed bell peppers from the oven and let them cool for a few minutes. Garnish with fresh parsley.

13. Serve the Quinoa and Vegetable Stuffed Bell Peppers as a flavorful and nutritious main course. They can be enjoyed on their own or paired with a side salad for a complete meal.

LENTIL SOUP WITH KALE AND CARROTS

Ingredients

- 1 tablespoon olive oil

- 1 onion, diced

- 2 cloves garlic, minced

- 2 carrots, diced

- 2 celery stalks, diced

- 1 cup dried green or brown lentils, rinsed

- 6 cups vegetable broth or water

- 1 bay leaf

- 1 teaspoon dried thyme

- 1 teaspoon ground cumin

- 1/2 teaspoon paprika

- Salt and pepper, to taste

- 2 cups chopped kale, stems removed

- Juice of 1 lemon

- Fresh parsley, chopped (for garnish)

Instructions

1. In a large pot or Dutch oven, heat the olive oil over medium heat. Add the diced onion and minced garlic, and sauté until the onion becomes translucent and fragrant.

2. Add the diced carrots and celery to the pot. Cook for about 5 minutes, or until the vegetables start to soften.

3. Stir in the rinsed lentils, vegetable broth or water, bay leaf, dried thyme, ground cumin, paprika, salt, and pepper. Bring the mixture to a boil.

4. Reduce the heat to low, cover the pot, and simmer for about 30-40 minutes, or until the lentils are tender.

5. Add the chopped kale to the soup and stir well. Cook for an additional 5 minutes, or until the kale is wilted.

6. Remove the pot from the heat and discard the bay leaf.

7. Stir in the lemon juice, adjusting the amount to taste.

8. Ladle the Lentil Soup with Kale and Carrots into bowls. Garnish with fresh parsley.

9. Serve the soup as a comforting and nourishing lunch or dinner option. It pairs well with crusty bread or a side salad.

Lentil Soup with Kale and Carrots is a hearty and wholesome dish, packed with protein, fiber, and a variety of nutrients. It's a perfect choicefor a satisfying and healthy meal. Enjoy!

Here are two more recipes for Tuna Salad Lettuce Wraps and Greek Salad with Grilled Chicken:

Tuna Salad Lettuce Wraps

Ingredients:

- 2 cans tuna, drained

- 1/4 cup mayonnaise (or Greek yogurt for a healthier option)

- 1 tablespoon Dijon mustard

- 1/4 cup diced red onion

- 1/4 cup diced celery

- 1/4 cup diced pickles (optional)

- 1 tablespoon lemon juice

- Salt and pepper, to taste

- Lettuce leaves (such as iceberg or romaine) for wrapping

- Sliced tomatoes and cucumber (optional, for serving)

Instructions

1. In a mixing bowl, combine the drained tuna, mayonnaise (or Greek yogurt), Dijon mustard, diced red onion, diced

celery, diced pickles (if using), lemon juice, salt, and pepper. Mix well until all the ingredients are evenly combined.

2. Taste the tuna salad and adjust the seasoning with additional salt, pepper, or lemon juice if desired.

3. Take a lettuce leaf and spoon a generous amount of the tuna salad onto the center of the leaf.

4. Fold the sides of the lettuce leaf over the filling, then roll it up tightly to create a wrap.

5. Repeat with the remaining lettuce leaves and tuna salad mixture.

6. Serve the Tuna Salad Lettuce Wraps with sliced tomatoes and cucumber on the side, if desired.

7. These lettuce wraps make a light and refreshing meal option, perfect for a quick lunch or a light dinner.

Greek Salad with Grilled Chicken

Ingredients:

For the grilled chicken:

- 2 boneless, skinless chicken breasts

- 2 tablespoons olive oil

- 2 cloves garlic, minced

- 1 teaspoon dried oregano

- Salt and pepper, to taste

For the Greek salad:

- 4 cups mixed salad greens

- 1 cup cherry tomatoes, halved

- 1 cucumber, diced

- 1/2 red onion, thinly sliced

- 1/2 cup Kalamata olives, pitted

- 1/2 cup crumbled feta cheese

- 1/4 cup chopped fresh parsley

- Juice of 1 lemon

- 2 tablespoons extra-virgin olive oil

- Salt and pepper, to taste

Instructions

1. Preheat the grill to medium-high heat.

2. In a bowl, combine the olive oil, minced garlic, dried oregano, salt, and pepper. Mix well.

3. Pat the chicken breasts dry and brush them with the olive oil mixture, coating both sides.

4. Place the chicken breasts on the preheated grill and cook for about 6-8 minutes per side, or until the internal temperature

reaches 165°F (74°C). Remove the chicken from the grill and let it rest for a few minutes before slicing.

5. In a large salad bowl, combine the mixed salad greens, cherry tomatoes, diced cucumber, thinly sliced red onion, Kalamata olives, crumbled feta cheese, and chopped fresh parsley.

6. In a small bowl, whisk together the lemon juice, extra-virgin olive oil, salt, and pepper to make the dressing.

7. Pour the dressing over the salad ingredients in the large mixing bowl and toss gently to coat everything evenly.

8. Slice the grilled chicken breasts into thin strips.

9. Divide the Greek salad among serving plates or bowls and top with the sliced grilled chicken.

10. Serve the Greek Salad with Grilled Chicken as a satisfying and flavorful meal. It can be enjoyed as a light lunch or dinner option.

Greek Salad with Grilled Chicken is a delicious and nutritious combination of fresh vegetables, tangy feta cheese, and grilled chicken. It's a perfect choice for a healthy and satisfying meal. Enjoy!

Here are two more recipes for Vegetable and Bean Chili and Hummus and Veggie Sandwich on Whole Grain Bread:

Vegetable and Bean Chili

Ingredients:

- 2 tablespoons olive oil

- 1 onion, diced

- 2 cloves garlic, minced

- 1 bell pepper, diced

- 1 zucchini, diced

- 1 carrot, diced

- 1 can diced tomatoes

- 1 can kidney beans, drained and rinsed

- 1 can black beans, drained and rinsed

- 1 cup corn kernels (fresh or frozen)

- 2 tablespoons chili powder

- 1 teaspoon ground cumin

- 1 teaspoon paprika

- 1/2 teaspoon dried oregano

- Salt and pepper, to taste

- Optional toppings: shredded cheese, sour cream, chopped fresh cilantro, diced avocado

Instructions

1. In a large pot or Dutch oven, heat the olive oil over medium heat.

2. Add the diced onion and minced garlic to the pot. Sauté until the onion becomes translucent and fragrant.

3. Add the diced bell pepper, zucchini, and carrot to the pot. Cook for about 5 minutes, or until the vegetables start to soften.

4. Stir in the diced tomatoes, kidney beans, black beans, corn kernels, chili powder, ground cumin, paprika, dried oregano, salt, and pepper. Mix well to combine all the ingredients.

5. Bring the chili to a boil, then reduce the heat to low. Cover the pot and let it simmer for at least 30 minutes to allow the flavors to meld together. You can simmer it for longer if desired, to enhance the flavor.

6. Taste the chili and adjust the seasoning with additional salt, pepper, or spices if needed.

7. Serve the Vegetable and Bean Chili hot, garnished with shredded cheese, sour cream, chopped fresh cilantro, and diced avocado if desired. It pairs well with crusty bread or cornbread.

HUMMUS AND VEGGIE SANDWICH ON WHOLE GRAIN BREAD

Ingredients:

- 4 slices whole grain bread

- 1/2 cup hummus (store-bought or homemade)

- 1 cucumber, thinly sliced

- 1 carrot, grated

- 1/2 red bell pepper, thinly sliced

- A handful of baby spinach or mixed greens

- Salt and pepper, to taste

Instructions:

1. Spread a generous amount of hummus on one side of each slice of whole grain bread.

2. Place a layer of cucumber slices on two slices of bread.

3. Top the cucumber with grated carrot, red bell pepper slices, and a handful of baby spinach or mixed greens.

4. Sprinkle salt and pepper over the vegetables to season to taste.

5. Place the remaining slices of bread, hummus-side down, on top of the vegetable layers.

6. Press the sandwich gently together.

7. Cut the sandwich in half or into quarters for easier handling, if desired.

8. Serve the Hummus and Veggie Sandwich as a healthy and satisfying meal. It's packed with fiber, vitamins, and minerals

from the vegetables and whole grain bread, while the hummus adds a creamy and flavorful element.

Both the Vegetable and Bean Chili and the Hummus and Veggie Sandwich offer nutritious and delicious options for meals. They are versatile, customizable, and can be enjoyed by vegetarians and non-vegetarians alike. These recipes are great for lunch or dinner and are sure to satisfy your hunger while providing a boost of energy and essential nutrients.

Broccoli and Quinoa Salad with Lemon Dressing

Here's a recipe for Broccoli and Quinoa Salad with Lemon Dressing:

Ingredients

- 1 cup quinoa

- 2 cups vegetable broth or water

- 2 cups broccoli florets

- 1/2 cup cherry tomatoes, halved

- 1/4 cup red onion, finely chopped

- 1/4 cup chopped fresh parsley

- 1/4 cup chopped fresh mint

- 1/4 cup crumbled feta cheese (optional)

- 1/4 cup sliced almonds, toasted

- Salt and pepper, to taste

For the Lemon Dressing:

- 3 tablespoons extra-virgin olive oil

- 2 tablespoons fresh lemon juice

- 1 teaspoon Dijon mustard

- 1 clove garlic, minced

- Salt and pepper, to taste

Instructions:

1. Rinse the quinoa under cold water to remove any bitterness.

2. In a saucepan, bring the vegetable broth or water to a boil. Add the quinoa, reduce the heat to low, cover, and simmer for about 15 minutes, or until the quinoa is tender and the liquid is absorbed.

3. Remove the cooked quinoa from heat and let it cool to room temperature.

4. Steam the broccoli florets until they are bright green and slightly tender, about 3-5 minutes. Immediately transfer the steamed broccoli to a bowl of ice water to stop the cooking process. Drain and set aside.

5. In a large salad bowl, combine the cooked and cooled quinoa, steamed broccoli florets, cherry tomatoes, red onion, chopped fresh parsley, chopped fresh mint, crumbled feta cheese (if using), and sliced almonds.

6. In a small bowl, whisk together the extra-virgin olive oil, fresh lemon juice, Dijon mustard, minced garlic, salt, and pepper to make the lemon dressing.

7. Pour the lemon dressing over the salad ingredients and toss gently to coat everything evenly.

8. Taste the salad and adjust the seasoning with additional salt, pepper, or lemon juice if desired.

9. Allow the flavors to meld together by refrigerating the salad for at least 30 minutes before serving.

10. Serve the Broccoli and Quinoa Salad with Lemon Dressing as a delicious and nutritious side dish or a light and satisfying main course.

This salad is packed with wholesome ingredients like quinoa, broccoli, tomatoes, and fresh herbs. The lemon dressing adds a bright and tangy flavor that complements the other ingredients perfectly. It's a great option for a healthy lunch or as a side dish for dinner. Enjoy!

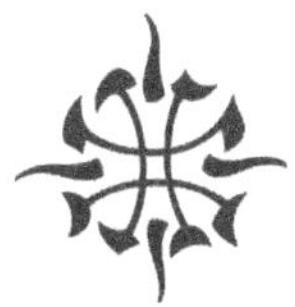

Chapter 4

Dinner Recipes

Baked Salmon with Dill and Lemon

Here's a recipe for Baked Salmon with Dill and Lemon:

Ingredients:

- 4 salmon fillets (about 6 ounces each)

- Salt and pepper, to taste

- 2 tablespoons fresh dill, chopped

- 2 tablespoons fresh lemon juice

- 2 tablespoons extra-virgin olive oil

- 2 cloves garlic, minced

- Lemon slices, for garnish

Instructions:

1. Preheat your oven to 375°F (190°C). Line a baking sheet with parchment paper or aluminum foil for easy cleanup.

2. Place the salmon fillets on the prepared baking sheet. Season both sides of the salmon with salt and pepper to taste.

3. In a small bowl, combine the fresh dill, fresh lemon juice, extra-virgin olive oil, and minced garlic. Stir well to make a marinade.

4. Pour the marinade over the salmon fillets, making sure to coat them evenly. You can use a brush or your hands to spread the marinade over the salmon.

5. Place a few lemon slices on top of each salmon fillet for additional flavor and presentation.

6. Bake the salmon in the preheated oven for about 12-15 minutes, or until the salmon is cooked through and flakes easily with a fork. The cooking time may vary depending on the thickness of the fillets, so keep an eye on them to avoid overcooking.

7. Once the salmon is cooked, remove it from the oven and let it rest for a few minutes.

8. Serve the Baked Salmon with Dill and Lemon hot. You can garnish it with additional fresh dill and lemon slices if desired.

This recipe creates moist and flavorful salmon with the zesty combination of dill and lemon. The marinade helps to infuse the salmon with delicious flavors and keeps it tender during baking. It's a healthy and delicious option for a main course that pairs well with a variety of side dishes such as roasted vegetables, quinoa, or a fresh green salad. Enjoy!

Here's a recipe for Grilled Chicken with Rosemary and Garlic, as well as a recipe for Spaghetti Squash Primavera:

Grilled Chicken with Rosemary and Garlic

Ingredients:

- 4 boneless, skinless chicken breasts

- 4 cloves garlic, minced

- 2 tablespoons fresh rosemary, chopped

- 2 tablespoons olive oil

- 1 tablespoon lemon juice

- Salt and pepper, to taste

Instructions:

1. Preheat your grill to medium-high heat.

2. In a small bowl, combine the minced garlic, chopped rosemary, olive oil, lemon juice, salt, and pepper. Mix well to create a marinade.

3. Place the chicken breasts in a shallow dish or resealable plastic bag. Pour the marinade over the chicken, making sure each breast is well coated. Allow the chicken to marinate for at least 30 minutes, or refrigerate for up to 4 hours for more flavor.

4. Remove the chicken from the marinade and discard any excess marinade.

5. Grill the chicken breasts on the preheated grill for about 6-8 minutes per side, or until the internal temperature reaches 165°F (74°C) and the chicken is cooked through.

6. Remove the chicken from the grill and let it rest for a few minutes before serving.

7. Serve the Grilled Chicken with Rosemary and Garlic hot. You can garnish with additional fresh rosemary sprigs if desired. It pairs well with a side of roasted vegetables, rice, or a fresh salad.

SPAGHETTI SQUASH PRIMAVERA

Ingredients:

- 1 medium spaghetti squash

- 2 tablespoons olive oil

- 2 cloves garlic, minced

- 1 small onion, diced

- 1 bell pepper, thinly sliced

- 1 small zucchini, diced

- 1 small yellow squash, diced

- 1 cup cherry tomatoes, halved

- 1/2 cup vegetable broth

- 1/4 cup grated Parmesan cheese (optional)

- Salt and pepper, to taste

- Fresh basil leaves, for garnish

Instructions:

1. Preheat your oven to 400°F (200°C).

2. Cut the spaghetti squash in half lengthwise and scoop out the seeds. Brush the cut sides of the squash with olive oil and sprinkle with salt and pepper.

3. Place the spaghetti squash halves, cut side down, on a baking sheet lined with parchment paper. Roast in the preheated oven for 40-50 minutes, or until the squash is tender and the strands can be easily separated with a fork.

4. While the squash is roasting, heat the olive oil in a large skillet over medium heat. Add the minced garlic and diced onion to the skillet. Sauté for 2-3 minutes, until fragrant and slightly softened.

5. Add the bell pepper, zucchini, and yellow squash to the skillet. Cook for an additional 5-7 minutes, or until the vegetables are crisp-tender.

6. Stir in the halved cherry tomatoes and vegetable broth. Cook for another 2-3 minutes, until the tomatoes are slightly softened.

7. Use a fork to scrape the cooked spaghetti squash strands into the skillet with the vegetables. Toss everything together to combine. Season with salt and pepper to taste.

8. If desired, sprinkle grated Parmesan cheese over the spaghetti squash primavera and stir to melt and incorporate.

9. Transfer the spaghetti squash primavera to serving plates or bowls. Garnish with fresh basil leaves.

10. Serve the Spaghetti Squash Primavera as a flavorful and healthy vegetarian main course. It can also be served as a side dish alongside grilled chicken or fish.

These recipes offer a delicious and nutritious combination for a satisfying meal. The Grilled Chicken with Rosemary and Garlic is packed with flavor from the marinade, while the Spaghetti Squash Primavera provides a colorful and veggie-packed dish. Enjoy!

Here's a recipe for Vegetable Stir-Fry with Tofu, as well as a recipe for Turkey Meatballs with Marinara Sauce:

VEGETABLE STIR-FRY WITH TOFU

Ingredients

- 14 ounces firm tofu, drained and cut into cubes

- 2 tablespoons soy sauce

- 1 tablespoon hoisin sauce

- 1 tablespoon rice vinegar

- 1 tablespoon sesame oil

- 1 tablespoon vegetable oil

- 2 cloves garlic, minced

- 1 inch ginger, grated

- 1 red bell pepper, sliced

- 1 yellow bell pepper, sliced

- 1 medium carrot, sliced

- 1 cup broccoli florets

- 1 cup snow peas

- 1 cup mushrooms, sliced

- Salt and pepper, to taste

- 2 green onions, sliced (for garnish)

- Sesame seeds (for garnish)

Instructions

1. In a small bowl, whisk together the soy sauce, hoisin sauce, rice vinegar, and sesame oil. Set aside.

2. Heat the vegetable oil in a large skillet or wok over medium-high heat. Add the minced garlic and grated ginger, and cook for about 1 minute until fragrant.

3. Add the tofu cubes to the skillet and cook until they are lightly browned on all sides, about 5 minutes. Remove the tofu from the skillet and set aside.

4. In the same skillet, add the sliced bell peppers, carrot, broccoli florets, snow peas, and mushrooms. Stir-fry the vegetables for about 5-7 minutes, or until they are crisp-tender.

5. Return the tofu to the skillet with the vegetables. Pour the sauce mixture over the tofu and vegetables, and toss to coat everything evenly. Cook for an additional 2-3 minutes, until the tofu is heated through.

6. Season the stir-fry with salt and pepper to taste.

7. Remove the skillet from the heat and garnish the stir-fry with sliced green onions and sesame seeds.

8. Serve the Vegetable Stir-Fry with Tofu hot over steamed rice or noodles for a healthy and flavorful meal.

Turkey Meatballs with Marinara Sauce

Ingredients:

For the meatballs:

- 1 pound ground turkey

- 1/2 cup breadcrumbs

- 1/4 cup grated Parmesan cheese

- 1/4 cup milk

- 1/4 cup finely chopped fresh parsley

- 1 egg, lightly beaten

- 2 cloves garlic, minced

- 1 teaspoon dried oregano

- 1/2 teaspoon salt

- 1/4 teaspoon black pepper

For the marinara sauce:

- 2 tablespoons olive oil

- 1 small onion, finely chopped

- 2 cloves garlic, minced

- 1 can (14 ounces) crushed tomatoes

- 1 can (14 ounces) diced tomatoes

- 1 teaspoon dried basil

- 1 teaspoon dried oregano

- 1/2 teaspoon sugar

- Salt and pepper, to taste

Instructions

1. Preheat your oven to 400°F (200°C). Line a baking sheet with parchment paper.

2. In a large mixing bowl, combine the ground turkey, breadcrumbs, grated Parmesan cheese, milk, chopped parsley, egg, minced garlic, dried oregano, salt, and black pepper. Mix well until all the ingredients are thoroughly combined.

3. Roll the mixture into meatballs, about 1 inch in diameter. Place the meatballs on the prepared baking sheet.

4. Bake the meatballs in the preheated oven for 20-25 minutes, or until they are cooked through and browned.

5. While the meatballs are baking, prepare the marinara sauce. Heat the olive oil in a large saucepan over medium heat. Add the chopped onion and minced garlic, and sauté until they are softened and fragrant.

6. Add the crushed tomatoes, diced tomatoes, dried basil, dried oregano, sugar, salt, and pepper to the saucepan. Stir well to combine.

7. Reduce the heat to low and simmer the sauce for about 15-20 minutes, allowing the flavors to meld together.

8. Once the meatballs are cooked, transfer them to the simmering marinara sauce. Gently stir to coat the meatballs with the sauce.

9. Continue to simmer the meatballs in the sauce for an additional 10-15 minutes, allowing the flavors to blend.

10. Serve the Turkey Meatballs with Marinara Sauce hot. They can be enjoyed on their own or served with pasta, rice, or crusty bread.

These recipes provide a delicious and satisfying combination of flavors. The Vegetable Stir-Fry with Tofu is loaded with colorful veggies and a tasty sauce, while the Turkey Meatballs with Marinara Sauce are tender and flavorful. Enjoy!

Absolutely! Here's a recipe for Roasted Vegetable Quinoa Bowl, as well as a recipe for Cauliflower Crust Pizza with Pesto and Cherry Tomatoes:

ROASTED VEGETABLE QUINOA BOWL

Ingredients:

- 1 cup quinoa

- 2 cups water or vegetable broth

- 1 small butternut squash, peeled and cubed

- 2 bell peppers, seeded and sliced

- 1 red onion, sliced

- 2 cups broccoli florets

- 2 tablespoons olive oil

- 1 teaspoon dried thyme

- 1 teaspoon dried rosemary

- Salt and pepper, to taste

- 1/4 cup chopped fresh parsley

- 1/4 cup crumbled feta cheese (optional)

- Lemon wedges, for serving

Instructions:

1. Preheat your oven to 400°F (200°C). Line a baking sheet with parchment paper.

2. In a fine-mesh sieve, rinse the quinoa under cold water. In a medium saucepan, bring the water or vegetable broth to a boil. Add the rinsed quinoa and reduce the heat to low. Cover and simmer for about 15-20 minutes, or until the quinoa is cooked and the liquid is absorbed. Fluff the quinoa with a fork and set aside.

3. In a large bowl, combine the cubed butternut squash, sliced bell peppers, sliced red onion, and broccoli florets. Drizzle with olive oil and sprinkle with dried thyme, dried rosemary, salt, and pepper. Toss everything together until the vegetables are well coated.

4. Spread the vegetables in a single layer on the prepared baking sheet. Roast in the preheated oven for about 25-30

minutes, or until the vegetables are tender and slightly caramelized.

5. In serving bowls, divide the cooked quinoa and roasted vegetables. Top with fresh parsley and crumbled feta cheese, if desired.

6. Serve the Roasted Vegetable Quinoa Bowl hot, with a squeeze of lemon juice for added brightness and flavor.

This recipe creates a wholesome and satisfying meal that is packed with nutritious vegetables and protein-rich quinoa. The roasted vegetables add a delightful caramelized flavor, and the combination of herbs and spices enhances the overall taste. Enjoy!

CAULIFLOWER CRUST PIZZA WITH PESTO AND CHERRY TOMATOES

Ingredients

For the cauliflower crust:

- 1 medium cauliflower head, florets only

- 1/2 cup shredded mozzarella cheese

- 1/4 cup grated Parmesan cheese

- 1 teaspoon dried oregano

- 1/2 teaspoon garlic powder

- 2 eggs, lightly beaten

- Salt and pepper, to taste

For the toppings:

- 1/4 cup basil pesto

- 1 cup cherry tomatoes, halved

- 1/4 cup shredded mozzarella cheese

- Fresh basil leaves, for garnish

Instructions

1. Preheat your oven to 425°F (220°C). Line a baking sheet with parchment paper.

2. Place the cauliflower florets in a food processor and pulse until they resemble fine rice-like grains.

3. Transfer the cauliflower rice to a microwave-safe bowl. Microwave on high for 4-5 minutes, or until the cauliflower is tender. Let it cool slightly.

4. Using a clean kitchen towel or cheesecloth, squeeze out any excess moisture from the cooked cauliflower.

5. In a mixing bowl, combine the squeezed cauliflower, shredded mozzarella cheese, grated Parmesan cheese, dried oregano, garlic powder, beaten eggs, salt, and pepper. Mix well to form a dough-like consistency.

6. Transfer the cauliflower dough onto the prepared baking sheet. Use your hands to shape it into a thin, round crust.

7. Bake the cauliflower crust in the preheated oven for about 15-20 minutes, or until it becomes golden and slightly crispy.

8. Remove the crust from the oven and spread the basil pesto evenly over the surface.

9. Sprinkle the halved cherry tomatoes and shredded mozzarella cheese over the pesto.

10. Return the pizza to the oven and bake for an additional 8-10 minutes, or until the cheese is melted and bubbly.

11. Garnish the Cauliflower Crust Pizza with fresh basil leaves.

12. Slice and serve the pizza hot, enjoying the delicious combination of flavors from the cauliflower crust, pesto, and juicy cherry tomatoes.

This recipe offers a healthier twist to traditional pizza by using a cauliflower crust. The crust is gluten-free and low in carbs, while still providing a satisfying and flavorful base for your favorite toppings. Enjoy a guilt-free pizza night with this delicious Cauliflower Crust Pizza with Pesto and Cherry Tomatoes!

Here are the recipes for Baked Cod with Mediterranean Salsa and Stuffed Portobello Mushrooms with Quinoa and Spinach:

BAKED COD WITH MEDITERRANEAN SALSA

Ingredients:

- 4 cod fillets

- Salt and pepper, to taste

- 2 tablespoons olive oil

- 2 cloves garlic, minced

- 1 teaspoon dried oregano

- 1 teaspoon dried basil

- 1 cup cherry tomatoes, halved

- 1/2 cup pitted Kalamata olives, sliced

- 1/4 cup chopped fresh parsley

- 2 tablespoons lemon juice

- Lemon wedges, for serving

Instructions:

1. Preheat your oven to 400°F (200°C). Line a baking sheet with parchment paper.

2. Season the cod fillets with salt and pepper on both sides. Place the fillets on the prepared baking sheet.

3. In a small bowl, whisk together the olive oil, minced garlic, dried oregano, and dried basil. Drizzle the mixture over the cod fillets, ensuring they are evenly coated.

4. In a separate bowl, combine the halved cherry tomatoes, sliced Kalamata olives, chopped parsley, and lemon juice. Toss everything together to make the Mediterranean salsa.

5. Spoon the Mediterranean salsa over the cod fillets, distributing it evenly.

6. Bake the cod in the preheated oven for about 12-15 minutes, or until the fish is cooked through and flakes easily with a fork.

7. Remove the baked cod from the oven and let it rest for a few minutes.

8. Serve the Baked Cod with Mediterranean Salsa hot, with lemon wedges on the side for an extra burst of citrus flavor.

This recipe provides a light and flavorful way to enjoy cod fish. The Mediterranean salsa adds a tangy and herbaceous element, complementing the delicate taste of the fish. It's a perfect dish for a healthy and satisfying meal.

STUFFED PORTOBELLO MUSHROOMS WITH QUINOA AND SPINACH

Ingredients:

- 4 large Portobello mushrooms, stems removed

- 1 cup cooked quinoa

- 1 cup fresh spinach, chopped

- 1/2 cup shredded mozzarella cheese

- 1/4 cup grated Parmesan cheese

- 2 cloves garlic, minced

- 2 tablespoons olive oil

- 1 teaspoon dried oregano

- Salt and pepper, to taste

- Fresh basil leaves, for garnish

Instructions:

1. Preheat your oven to 375°F (190°C). Line a baking sheet with parchment paper.

2. Place the Portobello mushrooms on the prepared baking sheet, gill side up.

3. In a large mixing bowl, combine the cooked quinoa, chopped spinach, shredded mozzarella cheese, grated Parmesan cheese, minced garlic, olive oil, dried oregano, salt, and pepper. Mix well until all the ingredients are evenly incorporated.

4. Divide the quinoa and spinach mixture among the Portobello mushrooms, filling the cavities generously.

5. Bake the stuffed mushrooms in the preheated oven for about 20-25 minutes, or until the mushrooms are tender and the cheese is melted and slightly golden.

6. Remove the stuffed mushrooms from the oven and let them cool for a few minutes.

7. Garnish the Stuffed Portobello Mushrooms with fresh basil leaves.

8. Serve the mushrooms warm as a main dish or as a side dish alongside a salad or roasted vegetables.

These Stuffed Portobello Mushrooms with Quinoa and Spinach are a delicious and satisfying vegetarian option. The combination of flavors and textures creates a savory and nutritious meal. Enjoy the hearty goodness of these stuffed mushrooms!

LENTIL AND SWEET POTATO SHEPHERD'S PIE

Here's a recipe for Lentil and Sweet Potato Shepherd's Pie:

Ingredients:

For the lentil filling:

- 1 cup green or brown lentils

- 3 cups vegetable broth or water

- 1 tablespoon olive oil

- 1 onion, diced

- 2 carrots, diced

- 2 celery stalks, diced

- 3 cloves garlic, minced

- 1 teaspoon dried thyme

- 1 teaspoon dried rosemary

- 1 can (14 ounces) diced tomatoes

- 1 cup frozen peas

- Salt and pepper, to taste

For the sweet potato topping:

- 3 large sweet potatoes, peeled and cubed

- 2 tablespoons butter or olive oil

- 1/4 cup milk or non-dairy milk

- Salt and pepper, to taste

Instructions:

1. In a saucepan, combine the lentils and vegetable broth (or water) and bring to a boil. Reduce the heat to low, cover, and simmer for about 20-25 minutes, or until the lentils are tender but not mushy. Drain any excess liquid and set aside.

2. In a large skillet, heat the olive oil over medium heat. Add the diced onion, carrots, and celery. Sauté for about 5-7 minutes, or until the vegetables are softened.

3. Add the minced garlic, dried thyme, and dried rosemary to the skillet. Cook for an additional minute until the herbs are fragrant.

4. Stir in the cooked lentils, diced tomatoes (with their juice), and frozen peas. Season with salt and pepper to taste. Simmer the lentil filling for about 5-10 minutes, allowing the flavors to meld together. Remove from heat and set aside.

5. Meanwhile, place the cubed sweet potatoes in a large pot and cover with water. Bring to a boil and cook for about 15-20 minutes, or until the sweet potatoes are fork-tender.

6. Drain the cooked sweet potatoes and return them to the pot. Add butter (or olive oil) and milk (or non-dairy milk) to the pot. Mash the sweet potatoes until smooth and creamy. Season with salt and pepper to taste.

7. Preheat your oven to 375°F (190°C).

8. Transfer the lentil filling to a baking dish and spread it evenly. Top with the mashed sweet potatoes, smoothing the surface with a spoon or spatula.

9. Bake the Lentil and Sweet Potato Shepherd's Pie in the preheated oven for about 25-30 minutes, or until the filling is bubbly and the sweet potato topping is lightly golden.

10. Remove the Shepherd's Pie from the oven and let it cool for a few minutes before serving.

This Lentil and Sweet Potato Shepherd's Pie is a hearty and nutritious vegetarian dish. The lentil filling provides protein and fiber, while the creamy sweet potato topping adds a touch of sweetness. Enjoy this comforting and delicious meal!

Chapter 5

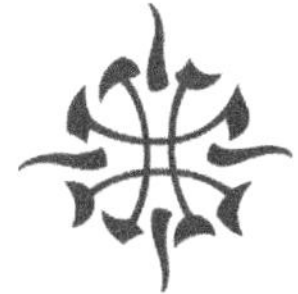

Snacks and Appetizers

GUACAMOLE WITH WHOLE GRAIN TORTILLA CHIPS

Here's a recipe for Guacamole with Whole Grain Tortilla Chips:

Ingredients

For the guacamole:

- 2 ripe avocados

- 1 small onion, finely diced

- 1 small tomato, seeded and diced

- 1 jalapeño pepper, seeded and minced (optional for heat)

- Juice of 1 lime

- 2 tablespoons chopped fresh cilantro

- Salt and pepper, to taste

For the whole grain tortilla chips:

- 4-6 whole grain tortillas

- Olive oil, for brushing

- Salt, to taste

Instructions:

1. Start by preparing the guacamole. Cut the avocados in half and remove the pits. Scoop out the flesh into a bowl.

2. Mash the avocado with a fork until desired consistency is reached (smooth or chunky).

3. Add the finely diced onion, diced tomato, minced jalapeño pepper (if using), lime juice, chopped cilantro, salt, and pepper to the mashed avocado. Mix well to combine all the ingredients.

4. Taste the guacamole and adjust the seasoning if needed. Add more lime juice, salt, or pepper to your preference.

5. Cover the guacamole with plastic wrap, ensuring that the wrap touches the surface of the guacamole to prevent browning. Refrigerate for at least 30 minutes to allow the flavors to meld together.

6. Preheat your oven to 350°F (175°C).

7. For the whole grain tortilla chips, brush each tortilla lightly with olive oil on both sides. Stack the tortillas and cut them into wedges using a sharp knife or a pizza cutter.

8. Arrange the tortilla wedges in a single layer on a baking sheet. Sprinkle with salt to taste.

9. Bake the tortilla chips in the preheated oven for about 10-12 minutes, or until they are golden brown and crispy. Keep an eye on them to prevent burning.

10. Remove the tortilla chips from the oven and let them cool slightly.

11. Serve the homemade guacamole with the crispy whole grain tortilla chips.

Enjoy the fresh and creamy flavors of homemade guacamole paired with the crunchy goodness of whole grain tortilla chips. It's a perfect appetizer or snack for any occasion!

Here are the recipes for Greek Yogurt Dip with Veggies and Trail Mix with Nuts and Dried Fruit:

GREEK YOGURT DIP WITH VEGGIES

Ingredients:

- 1 cup Greek yogurt

- 1 tablespoon lemon juice

- 1 clove garlic, minced

- 1 tablespoon chopped fresh dill (or 1 teaspoon dried dill)

- Salt and pepper, to taste

- Assorted fresh vegetables (e.g., cucumber slices, carrot sticks, bell pepper strips) for dipping

Instructions

1. In a bowl, combine the Greek yogurt, lemon juice, minced garlic, chopped fresh dill, salt, and pepper. Mix well until all the ingredients are thoroughly combined.

2. Taste the dip and adjust the seasoning if needed. Add more lemon juice, salt, or pepper according to your preference.

3. Cover the bowl with plastic wrap and refrigerate for at least 30 minutes to allow the flavors to meld together.

4. Wash and prepare the fresh vegetables for dipping by slicing them into sticks or manageable pieces.

5. Serve the Greek Yogurt Dip with the prepared fresh vegetables on a platter or in individual bowls. Enjoy!

This Greek Yogurt Dip is a healthy and refreshing option for a snack or appetizer. The creamy and tangy flavors of the yogurt combined with the fresh herbs make it a delicious accompaniment to crunchy vegetables.

TRAIL MIX WITH NUTS AND DRIED FRUIT

Ingredients:

- 1 cup mixed nuts (e.g., almonds, cashews, walnuts)

- 1 cup dried fruit (e.g., raisins, cranberries, apricots, goji berries)

- 1/2 cup seeds (e.g., pumpkin seeds, sunflower seeds)

- 1/2 cup dark chocolate chips or chunks (optional)

Instructions

1. In a mixing bowl, combine the mixed nuts, dried fruit, and seeds. Mix well to distribute the ingredients evenly.

2. If desired, add dark chocolate chips or chunks to the mixture. This is optional but adds a sweet and indulgent element to the trail mix.

3. Toss all the ingredients together until they are well combined.

4. Transfer the trail mix to an airtight container or individual snack bags for easy portioning and storage.

5. Enjoy the trail mix as a quick and nutritious snack on the go, or pack it in your lunchbox for a satisfying treat.

This Trail Mix with Nuts and Dried Fruit is a versatile and portable snack that provides a good balance of healthy fats, protein, and natural sugars. Feel free to customize it with your favorite nuts, dried fruits, and seeds for a personalized blend.

Certainly! Here are the recipes for Apple Slices with Almond Butter and Cottage Cheese and Pineapple:

APPLE SLICES WITH ALMOND BUTTER

Ingredients:

- 2 apples (any variety), cored and sliced

- Almond butter

Instructions:

1. Wash and core the apples. Slice them into thin, round slices.

2. Spread almond butter on one side of each apple slice. You can spread a thin layer or add more almond butter according to your preference.

3. Arrange the apple slices on a serving plate and serve immediately.

Enjoy the combination of crisp apple slices and creamy almond butter. This snack is not only delicious but also provides a good balance of natural sweetness, fiber, and healthy fats.

COTTAGE CHEESE AND PINEAPPLE

Ingredients:

- 1 cup cottage cheese

- 1 cup diced fresh pineapple

Instructions:

1. In a bowl, scoop out the cottage cheese.

2. Dice fresh pineapple into small pieces.

3. Add the diced pineapple to the bowl of cottage cheese.

4. Gently mix the cottage cheese and pineapple together until well combined.

5. Serve the cottage cheese and pineapple mixture as is, or you can refrigerate it for a short time to chill and enhance the flavors.

The combination of creamy cottage cheese and juicy pineapple creates a refreshing and satisfying snack. It's a great source of protein, vitamins, and minerals. Enjoy it as a light and nutritious option!

Here are the recipes for Hummus with Carrot and Celery Sticks and Whole Grain Crackers with Tuna Salad:

HUMMUS WITH CARROT AND CELERY STICKS

Ingredients:

- 1 cup canned chickpeas, drained and rinsed

- 2 tablespoons tahini

- 2 tablespoons lemon juice

- 1 clove garlic, minced

- 2 tablespoons olive oil

- Salt and pepper, to taste

- Carrot sticks

- Celery sticks

Instructions

1. In a food processor or blender, combine the chickpeas, tahini, lemon juice, minced garlic, olive oil, salt, and pepper.

2. Process the ingredients until smooth and creamy. If the hummus is too thick, you can add a tablespoon of water or more olive oil to reach your desired consistency. Taste and adjust the seasoning if needed.

3. Transfer the hummus to a serving bowl.

4. Wash and peel the carrots. Cut them into sticks.

5. Wash and cut the celery stalks into sticks as well.

6. Arrange the carrot and celery sticks around the bowl of hummus.

7. Serve the hummus with the carrot and celery sticks for dipping.

This classic combination of hummus with carrot and celery sticks provides a healthy and flavorful snack. The creamy hummus pairs perfectly with the crisp and refreshing vegetables, making it a satisfying and nutritious option.

Whole Grain Crackers with Tuna Salad

Ingredients

- 1 can (5 ounces) tuna, drained

- 2 tablespoons mayonnaise

- 1 tablespoon lemon juice

- 1 tablespoon chopped fresh parsley (optional)

- Salt and pepper, to taste

- Whole grain crackers

Instructions

1. In a bowl, flake the drained tuna using a fork.

2. Add mayonnaise, lemon juice, chopped fresh parsley (if using), salt, and pepper to the tuna. Mix well until all the ingredients are combined.

3. Taste the tuna salad and adjust the seasoning if needed. Add more lemon juice, salt, or pepper according to your preference.

4. Place a spoonful of the tuna salad on each whole grain cracker.

5. Arrange the tuna salad-topped crackers on a serving platter.

6. Serve the whole grain crackers with tuna salad as an appetizer or snack.

This simple and delicious snack of whole grain crackers topped with tuna salad provides a good source of protein and healthy fats. It's a convenient and satisfying option for a quick bite or party appetizer.

Here are the recipes for Baked Sweet Potato Fries and Edamame with Sea Salt:

BAKED SWEET POTATO FRIES

Ingredients:

- 2 large sweet potatoes

- 2 tablespoons olive oil

- 1 teaspoon paprika

- 1/2 teaspoon garlic powder

- 1/2 teaspoon salt

- 1/4 teaspoon black pepper

Instructions:

1. Preheat your oven to 425°F (220°C). Line a baking sheet with parchment paper or lightly grease it.

2. Wash and peel the sweet potatoes. Cut them into long, thin strips resembling fries.

3. In a large bowl, combine the sweet potato strips, olive oil, paprika, garlic powder, salt, and black pepper. Toss until the sweet potato fries are evenly coated with the seasoning mixture.

4. Spread the sweet potato fries in a single layer on the prepared baking sheet, making sure they are not overcrowded.

5. Bake in the preheated oven for about 20-25 minutes, flipping halfway through, until the fries are golden brown and crispy.

6. Remove the sweet potato fries from the oven and let them cool slightly before serving.

Enjoy the baked sweet potato fries as a healthier alternative to traditional fries. The natural sweetness of the sweet potatoes combined with the savory seasonings makes them a delicious and satisfying snack or side dish.

EDAMAME WITH SEA SALT

Ingredients:

- 2 cups frozen edamame (in pods)

- Sea salt, to taste

Instructions:

1. Bring a pot of water to a boil. Add a pinch of salt to the boiling water.

2. Add the frozen edamame pods to the boiling water and cook for about 3-5 minutes, or until the pods are tender.

3. Drain the cooked edamame pods and transfer them to a serving bowl.

4. Sprinkle sea salt over the edamame pods while they are still warm. Toss gently to coat the pods evenly with the salt.

5. Serve the edamame with sea salt as a snack or appetizer.

Edamame is a popular and nutritious snack that is rich in protein, fiber, and essential nutrients. The simple addition of sea salt enhances the natural flavors of the edamame pods, making them a delicious and satisfying option for a healthy snack.

Enjoy the Baked Sweet Potato Fries and Edamame with Sea Salt as flavorful and nutritious snacks or side dishes. They are both simple to prepare and provide a delightful combination of tastes and textures.

AVOCADO AND TOMATO BRUSCHETTA

Here's the recipe for Avocado and Tomato Bruschetta:

Ingredients:

- 1 baguette, sliced into ½-inch thick slices

- 2 ripe avocados

- 1 cup cherry tomatoes, halved

- 1 clove garlic, minced

- 2 tablespoons red onion, finely chopped

- 2 tablespoons fresh basil, chopped

- 1 tablespoon fresh lemon juice

- 2 tablespoons extra virgin olive oil

- Salt and pepper, to taste

Instructions:

1. Preheat your oven to 375°F (190°C). Place the baguette slices on a baking sheet and drizzle them with a little olive oil. Bake in the preheated oven for about 10 minutes, or until the slices are crispy and golden brown. Remove from the oven and set aside.

2. In a bowl, mash the ripe avocados with a fork until they reach your desired consistency. Add the minced garlic, chopped red onion, lemon juice, and chopped basil. Mix well to combine.

3. Gently fold in the halved cherry tomatoes into the avocado mixture. Season with salt and pepper to taste.

4. Drizzle the avocado and tomato mixture with extra virgin olive oil and give it a final gentle mix.

5. Spoon the avocado and tomato mixture onto each toasted baguette slice, spreading it evenly.

6. Arrange the bruschetta on a serving platter and garnish with additional fresh basil leaves if desired.

7. Serve the avocado and tomato bruschetta immediately as an appetizer or snack.

The Avocado and Tomato Bruschetta offers a delightful combination of creamy avocado, juicy tomatoes, and aromatic herbs. The crispy baguette slices provide a perfect contrast in texture. Enjoy this refreshing and flavorful dish!

BERRY AND YOGURT POPSICLES

Ingredients:

- 1 cup mixed berries (such as strawberries, blueberries, raspberries)

- 1 cup Greek yogurt

- 2 tablespoons honey (optional, for sweetness)

- Popsicle molds

- Popsicle sticks

Instructions

1. Wash and prepare the mixed berries by removing any stems or hulls. You can choose to leave them whole or chop them into smaller pieces, depending on your preference.

2. In a bowl, combine the Greek yogurt and honey (if using). Mix well until the honey is fully incorporated into the yogurt.

3. Add the mixed berries to the yogurt mixture. Gently fold and stir until the berries are evenly distributed throughout the yogurt.

4. Spoon the mixture into popsicle molds, filling them almost to the top. Leave a little space at the top for expansion as the popsicles freeze.

5. Insert popsicle sticks into each mold, making sure they are centered and secure.

6. Place the popsicle molds in the freezer and let them freeze for at least 4-6 hours, or until the popsicles are completely frozen.

7. Once the popsicles are frozen, remove them from the molds by running warm water over the molds for a few seconds. Gently pull the popsicles out.

8. Serve the Berry and Yogurt Popsicles immediately, or you can store them in an airtight container in the freezer for later enjoyment.

These Berry and Yogurt Popsicles are a refreshing and healthy treat that combines the natural sweetness of mixed berries with creamy Greek yogurt. They are perfect for cooling down on a hot day or as a guilt-free dessert option. Enjoy!

Certainly! Here are the recipes for Dark Chocolate Covered Almonds and Frozen Banana Bites with Peanut Butter:

Dark Chocolate Covered Almonds

Ingredients:

- 1 cup whole almonds

- 8 ounces dark chocolate, chopped

- Optional toppings: sea salt, shredded coconut, crushed nuts

Instructions:

1. Line a baking sheet with parchment paper.

2. In a microwave-safe bowl or using a double boiler, melt the dark chocolate until smooth and fully melted.

3. Add the whole almonds to the melted chocolate. Stir until the almonds are fully coated.

4. Using a fork or a slotted spoon, remove the chocolate-coated almonds from the bowl, allowing any excess chocolate to drip off.

5. Place the coated almonds on the prepared baking sheet, spacing them apart.

6. If desired, sprinkle the coated almonds with a pinch of sea salt, shredded coconut, or crushed nuts while the chocolate is still wet.

7. Allow the chocolate to set by placing the baking sheet in the refrigerator for about 15-20 minutes, or until the chocolate is firm.

8. Once the chocolate is fully set, remove the dark chocolate-covered almonds from the refrigerator and transfer them to an airtight container or serving dish.

Enjoy these delicious and satisfying Dark Chocolate Covered Almonds as an indulgent treat or a homemade gift. The combination of rich dark chocolate and crunchy almonds is irresistible.

Frozen Banana Bites with Peanut Butter

Ingredients

- 2 large bananas, ripe but firm

- ¼ cup peanut butter

- Optional toppings: chopped nuts, shredded coconut, chocolate chips

Instructions:

1. Peel the bananas and slice them into ½-inch thick rounds.

2. Spread a small amount of peanut butter onto one side of each banana slice.

3. If desired, sprinkle the peanut butter with toppings such as chopped nuts, shredded coconut, or chocolate chips.

4. Place the banana slices on a baking sheet lined with parchment paper.

5. Transfer the baking sheet to the freezer and let the banana bites freeze for at least 2-3 hours, or until they are firm.

6. Once the banana bites are frozen, remove them from the baking sheet and transfer them to an airtight container or freezer bag for storage.

Enjoy these Frozen Banana Bites with Peanut Butter as a delightful and healthier dessert option. The creamy peanut butter pairs perfectly with the sweetness of the frozen banana, creating a satisfying and cooling treat.

Certainly! Here are the recipes for Greek Yogurt Bark with Berries and Nuts and Baked Apple Slices with Cinnamon:

GREEK YOGURT BARK WITH BERRIES AND NUTS

Ingredients:

- 1 cup Greek yogurt

- 2 tablespoons honey or maple syrup

- 1 teaspoon vanilla extract

- ½ cup mixed berries (such as blueberries, raspberries, and strawberries), chopped

- ¼ cup nuts (such as almonds, walnuts, or pistachios), chopped

- Optional: additional honey or maple syrup for drizzling

Instructions:

1. In a bowl, mix together the Greek yogurt, honey or maple syrup, and vanilla extract until well combined.

2. Line a baking sheet or tray with parchment paper.

3. Pour the Greek yogurt mixture onto the lined baking sheet, spreading it out evenly to create a thin layer.

4. Sprinkle the chopped berries and nuts over the yogurt, pressing them gently into the surface.

5. Optional: Drizzle some additional honey or maple syrup over the top for added sweetness.

6. Place the baking sheet in the freezer and let it freeze for at least 2-3 hours, or until the yogurt is completely frozen.

7. Once frozen, remove the Greek yogurt bark from the freezer and break it into pieces.

8. Serve the Greek Yogurt Bark with Berries and Nuts immediately or store it in an airtight container in the freezer for later enjoyment.

This Greek Yogurt Bark with Berries and Nuts is a delicious and nutritious dessert or snack option. The creamy Greek yogurt provides a tangy base, while the combination of sweet berries and crunchy nuts adds texture and flavor.

Baked Apple Slices with Cinnamon

Ingredients:

- 2 large apples, cored and thinly sliced

- 1 tablespoon melted butter or coconut oil

- 1 tablespoon honey or maple syrup

- 1 teaspoon ground cinnamon

- Optional toppings: chopped nuts, raisins, or a drizzle of caramel sauce

Instructions:

1. Preheat your oven to 350°F (175°C). Line a baking sheet with parchment paper.

2. In a bowl, combine the melted butter or coconut oil, honey or maple syrup, and ground cinnamon. Mix until well combined.

3. Add the apple slices to the bowl and toss them gently in the mixture until evenly coated.

4. Arrange the coated apple slices in a single layer on the lined baking sheet.

5. Optional: Sprinkle some chopped nuts or raisins over the apple slices for added flavor and texture.

6. Bake in the preheated oven for about 15-20 minutes, or until the apple slices are tender and slightly caramelized.

7. Remove the baked apple slices from the oven and let them cool slightly.

8. Serve the Baked Apple Slices with Cinnamon as a warm and comforting dessert. You can enjoy them on their own or pair them with a scoop of vanilla ice cream or a drizzle of caramel sauce if desired.

These Baked Apple Slices with Cinnamon are a delightful and healthier twist on a classic dessert. The warmth of the cinnamon combined with the natural sweetness of the baked apples creates a cozy and satisfying treat.

Here are the recipes for Oatmeal Raisin Cookies with Whole Grain Flour and Chia Seed and Berry Jam Thumbprint Cookies:

OATMEAL RAISIN COOKIES WITH WHOLE GRAIN FLOUR

Ingredients:

- 1 cup whole grain flour (such as whole wheat or spelt flour)

- 1 cup rolled oats

- 1/2 teaspoon baking soda

- 1/2 teaspoon ground cinnamon

- 1/4 teaspoon salt

- 1/2 cup unsalted butter, softened

- 1/2 cup brown sugar

- 1/4 cup granulated sugar

- 1 large egg

- 1 teaspoon vanilla extract

- 1/2 cup raisins

Instructions:

1. Preheat your oven to 350°F (175°C). Line a baking sheet with parchment paper.

2. In a medium bowl, whisk together the whole grain flour, rolled oats, baking soda, cinnamon, and salt. Set aside.

3. In a separate large bowl, cream together the softened butter, brown sugar, and granulated sugar until light and fluffy.

4. Add the egg and vanilla extract to the butter and sugar mixture. Beat until well combined.

5. Gradually add the dry ingredient mixture to the wet mixture, stirring until just combined.

6. Stir in the raisins until evenly distributed throughout the cookie dough.

7. Drop rounded spoonfuls of the cookie dough onto the prepared baking sheet, spacing them about 2 inches apart.

8. Bake in the preheated oven for 10-12 minutes, or until the edges are golden brown.

9. Remove the cookies from the oven and let them cool on the baking sheet for a few minutes before transferring them to a wire rack to cool completely.

10. Once cooled, store the Oatmeal Raisin Cookies in an airtight container for up to a week.

These Oatmeal Raisin Cookies with Whole Grain Flour are a wholesome and delicious treat. The combination of hearty whole grain flour, chewy oats, and sweet raisins makes for a satisfying cookie with a hint of cinnamon.

CHIA SEED AND BERRY JAM THUMBPRINT COOKIES

Ingredients:

- 1 cup all-purpose flour

- 1/2 cup unsalted butter, softened

- 1/4 cup granulated sugar

- 1 teaspoon vanilla extract

- 2 tablespoons chia seeds

- 1/4 cup berry jam or preserves (such as strawberry or raspberry)

Instructions:

1. Preheat your oven to 350°F (175°C). Line a baking sheet with parchment paper.

2. In a bowl, cream together the softened butter, granulated sugar, and vanilla extract until light and fluffy.

3. Gradually add the flour to the butter mixture, mixing until a soft dough forms.

4. Stir in the chia seeds until evenly distributed throughout the dough.

5. Roll the dough into small balls, about 1 inch in diameter. Place them on the prepared baking sheet, spacing them about 2 inches apart.

6. Use your thumb or the back of a spoon to make an indentation in the center of each cookie.

7. Spoon a small amount of berry jam or preserves into each indentation, filling it to the top.

8. Bake in the preheated oven for 10-12 minutes, or until the edges of the cookies are golden brown.

9. Remove the cookies from the oven and let them cool on the baking sheet for a few minutes before transferring them to a wire rack to cool completely.

10. Once cooled, store the Chia Seed and Berry Jam Thumbprint Cookies in an airtight container for up to a week.

These Chia Seed and Berry Jam Thumbprint Cookies are a delightful twist on the classic thumbprint cookie. The addition of chia seeds adds a nutritional boost, while the sweet and tangy berry jam creates a burst of flavor in every bite.

Certainly! Here are the recipes for Banana Bread with Walnuts and Mixed Berry Crisp with Oat Topping:

BANANA BREAD WITH WALNUTS

Ingredients:

- 2 cups all-purpose flour

- 1 teaspoon baking soda

- 1/2 teaspoon salt

- 1/2 teaspoon ground cinnamon

- 1/4 teaspoon ground nutmeg

- 1/2 cup unsalted butter, softened

- 3/4 cup granulated sugar

- 2 large eggs

- 3 ripe bananas, mashed

- 1 teaspoon vanilla extract

- 1/2 cup chopped walnuts

Instructions:

1. Preheat your oven to 350°F (175°C). Grease a loaf pan with butter or cooking spray.

2. In a bowl, whisk together the flour, baking soda, salt, cinnamon, and nutmeg. Set aside.

3. In a separate large bowl, cream together the softened butter and granulated sugar until light and fluffy.

4. Add the eggs, mashed bananas, and vanilla extract to the butter and sugar mixture. Beat until well combined.

5. Gradually add the dry ingredient mixture to the wet mixture, stirring until just combined. Do not overmix.

6. Fold in the chopped walnuts.

7. Pour the batter into the greased loaf pan, spreading it out evenly.

8. Bake in the preheated oven for 50-60 minutes, or until a toothpick inserted into the center of the bread comes out clean.

9. Remove the banana bread from the oven and let it cool in the pan for about 10 minutes. Then, transfer it to a wire rack to cool completely.

10. Once cooled, slice the Banana Bread with Walnuts and serve. It can be stored in an airtight container at room temperature for a few days.

This Banana Bread with Walnuts is a classic and comforting treat. The ripe bananas add natural sweetness and moisture, while the walnuts provide a delicious crunch and nutty flavor.

MIXED BERRY CRISP WITH OAT TOPPING

Ingredients:

- 4 cups mixed berries (such as strawberries, blueberries, raspberries, and blackberries)

- 1/4 cup granulated sugar

- 1 tablespoon cornstarch

- 1 tablespoon lemon juice

- 1 cup old-fashioned oats

- 1/2 cup all-purpose flour

- 1/2 cup packed brown sugar

- 1/2 teaspoon ground cinnamon

- 1/4 teaspoon salt

- 1/2 cup unsalted butter, melted

Instructions:

1. Preheat your oven to 350°F (175°C). Grease a baking dish with butter or cooking spray.

2. In a bowl, combine the mixed berries, granulated sugar, cornstarch, and lemon juice. Toss until the berries are evenly coated. Pour the berry mixture into the prepared baking dish.

3. In a separate bowl, mix together the oats, flour, brown sugar, cinnamon, and salt.

4. Pour the melted butter over the oat mixture and stir until it is evenly combined and crumbly.

5. Sprinkle the oat topping evenly over the berries in the baking dish.

6. Bake in the preheated oven for 30-35 minutes, or until the fruit is bubbling and the topping is golden brown.

7. Remove the mixed berry crisp from the oven and let it cool for a few minutes before serving.

8. Serve the Mixed Berry Crisp with Oat Topping warm, either on its own or with a scoop of vanilla ice cream or a dollop of whipped cream.

This Mixed Berry Crisp with Oat Topping is a delightful and fruity dessert. The combination of sweet and tart mixed berries with the crunchy and buttery oat topping creates a delicious contrast of flavors and textures.

Pumpkin Spice Energy Bites

Here's a recipe for Pumpkin Spice Energy Bites:

Ingredients:

- 1 cup rolled oats

- 1/2 cup pumpkin puree

- 1/4 cup almond butter or any nut butter of your choice

- 1/4 cup honey or maple syrup

- 1/4 cup ground flaxseed

- 1/4 cup chopped nuts (such as walnuts or pecans)

- 1/4 cup dried cranberries or raisins

- 1 teaspoon pumpkin spice blend

- 1/2 teaspoon vanilla extract

- Pinch of salt

- Optional: shredded coconut or additional oats for rolling

Instructions:

1. In a large bowl, combine the rolled oats, pumpkin puree, almond butter, honey or maple syrup, ground flaxseed, chopped nuts, dried cranberries or raisins, pumpkin spice blend, vanilla extract, and a pinch of salt.

2. Stir all the ingredients together until well combined. The mixture should be sticky and hold together.

3. Place the bowl in the refrigerator for about 15-20 minutes to allow the mixture to firm up slightly.

4. Once chilled, remove the bowl from the refrigerator. Take small portions of the mixture and roll them into bite-sized balls using your hands.

5. Optional: If desired, roll the energy bites in shredded coconut or additional oats for extra texture.

6. Place the energy bites on a baking sheet lined with parchment paper or a silicone mat.

7. Repeat the rolling process until all the mixture is used.

8. Place the energy bites in the refrigerator for at least 30 minutes to set and firm up.

9. Once set, transfer the Pumpkin Spice Energy Bites to an airtight container and store them in the refrigerator for up to a week.

These Pumpkin Spice Energy Bites are a delicious and nutritious snack option. Packed with oats, pumpkin, nuts, and spices, they provide a burst of energy and the flavors of fall. Enjoy them as a quick pick-me-up during the day or as a pre- or post-workout snack.

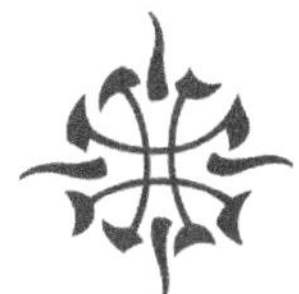

Chapter 7

Beverages and Drinks

Green Tea with Lemon and Honey

Here's a recipe for Green Tea with Lemon and Honey:

Ingredients:

- 1 green tea bag

- 1 cup hot water

- 1 tablespoon freshly squeezed lemon juice

- 1 teaspoon honey (adjust to taste)

Instructions:

1. Place the green tea bag in a cup.

2. Pour hot water over the tea bag and let it steep for 2-3 minutes, or according to the instructions on the tea bag packaging.

3. Once the tea has steeped, remove the tea bag and discard it.

4. Stir in the freshly squeezed lemon juice into the brewed green tea.

5. Add honey to the tea and stir until it is dissolved. Adjust the amount of honey according to your desired sweetness.

6. Taste the tea and add more lemon juice or honey if desired.

7. Serve the Green Tea with Lemon and Honey hot and enjoy!

Green Tea with Lemon and Honey is a refreshing and soothing beverage that combines the health benefits of green tea with the tangy brightness of lemon and the natural sweetness of honey. It's a perfect drink to enjoy in the morning or throughout the day.

Here are the recipes for a Berry Smoothie with Spinach and Coconut Water with Pineapple and Mint:

BERRY SMOOTHIE WITH SPINACH

Ingredients:

- 1 cup mixed berries (such as strawberries, blueberries, and raspberries)

- 1 ripe banana

- 1 cup fresh spinach leaves

- 1/2 cup plain Greek yogurt

- 1/2 cup almond milk (or any milk of your choice)

- 1 tablespoon honey or maple syrup (optional, for added sweetness)

- Ice cubes (optional, for a colder smoothie)

Instructions:

1. Place all the ingredients (mixed berries, ripe banana, fresh spinach leaves, Greek yogurt, almond milk, and honey or maple syrup) into a blender.

2. Blend on high speed until the mixture is smooth and creamy. If desired, add ice cubes and blend again until the smoothie is chilled.

3. Taste the smoothie and adjust the sweetness by adding more honey or maple syrup if desired.

4. Pour the Berry Smoothie with Spinach into glasses and serve immediately.

This Berry Smoothie with Spinach is a nutritious and delicious way to start your day or enjoy as a refreshing snack. The combination of sweet berries, creamy banana, nutrient-rich spinach, and protein-packed Greek yogurt creates a well-balanced and satisfying smoothie.

COCONUT WATER WITH PINEAPPLE AND MINT

Ingredients:

- 1 cup coconut water

- 1 cup pineapple chunks (fresh or frozen)

- 4-5 fresh mint leaves

- Ice cubes (optional, for a colder drink)

Instructions:

1. In a blender, combine the coconut water, pineapple chunks, and fresh mint leaves.

2. Blend on high speed until the mixture is smooth and well combined.

3. If desired, add ice cubes to the blender and blend again until the drink is chilled.

4. Taste the coconut water with pineapple and mint and adjust the sweetness or mint flavor if desired.

5. Pour the Coconut Water with Pineapple and Mint into glasses and serve immediately.

This Coconut Water with Pineapple and Mint is a refreshing and hydrating beverage with a tropical twist. The natural sweetness of pineapple combined with the refreshing flavor of mint and the electrolyte-rich coconut water creates a revitalizing drink that's perfect for warm days or as a post-workout refresher.

Certainly! Here are the recipes for Turmeric Golden Milk Latte and Cucumber Mint Infused Water:

Turmeric Golden Milk Latte

Ingredients:

- 1 cup milk (dairy or plant-based)

- 1/2 teaspoon ground turmeric

- 1/4 teaspoon ground cinnamon

- 1/4 teaspoon ground ginger

- 1/4 teaspoon vanilla extract

- 1 teaspoon honey or maple syrup (adjust to taste)

- Pinch of black pepper (optional)

Instructions:

1. In a small saucepan, heat the milk over medium-low heat until it starts to steam. Do not allow it to boil.

2. Add the ground turmeric, ground cinnamon, ground ginger, and vanilla extract to the saucepan. Whisk well to combine the ingredients.

3. Continue to heat the mixture for about 3-5 minutes, stirring occasionally, until the flavors are well blended and the latte is hot.

4. If desired, add honey or maple syrup to sweeten the latte. Adjust the amount to your taste preferences.

5. If using, add a pinch of black pepper. Black pepper is known to enhance the absorption of curcumin, the active compound in turmeric.

6. Once the latte is well heated and all the ingredients are combined, remove the saucepan from the heat.

7. Pour the Turmeric Golden Milk Latte into a mug and serve hot.

This Turmeric Golden Milk Latte is a warm and comforting drink that features the health benefits of turmeric and warming spices. It's a great option for a cozy beverage any time of the day.

Cucumber Mint Infused Water

Ingredients:

- 1 medium cucumber, thinly sliced

- 8-10 fresh mint leaves

- Water

Instructions:

1. In a pitcher or a large jar, add the thinly sliced cucumber and fresh mint leaves.

2. Fill the pitcher or jar with water.

3. Stir gently to combine the ingredients and release the flavors.

4. Cover the pitcher or jar and place it in the refrigerator for at least 1-2 hours, or overnight, to allow the flavors to infuse into the water.

5. Once infused, strain the water if desired, or simply pour it into glasses with the cucumber and mint.

6. Serve the Cucumber Mint Infused Water chilled, either on its own or over ice cubes.

This Cucumber Mint Infused Water is a refreshing and hydrating beverage with a subtle hint of cucumber and mint. It's a great way to stay hydrated and add a touch of flavor to your water, especially during hot summer days or as a refreshing detox drink.

Certainly! Here are the recipes for Herbal Iced Tea with Citrus and Beetroot and Berry Juice:

HERBAL ICED TEA WITH CITRUS

Ingredients:

- 4 herbal tea bags (such as chamomile, peppermint, or hibiscus)

- 4 cups boiling water

- 1-2 tablespoons honey or maple syrup (adjust to taste)

- Juice of 1 lemon

- Juice of 1 orange

- Slices of lemon and orange for garnish

- Ice cubes

Instructions:

1. Place the herbal tea bags in a heatproof pitcher or jar.

2. Pour the boiling water over the tea bags and let it steep for about 5-10 minutes, or according to the instructions on the tea bag packaging.

3. After steeping, remove the tea bags and discard them.

4. Stir in honey or maple syrup into the brewed herbal tea until it is dissolved. Adjust the sweetness according to your taste.

5. Add the juice of one lemon and one orange into the pitcher and stir to combine.

6. Allow the tea to cool to room temperature, then place it in the refrigerator to chill for at least 1-2 hours.

7. Once chilled, fill glasses with ice cubes and pour the Herbal Iced Tea with Citrus into the glasses.

8. Garnish each glass with slices of lemon and orange.

9. Serve the Herbal Iced Tea with Citrus and enjoy!

This Herbal Iced Tea with Citrus is a refreshing and flavorful drink that combines the benefits of herbal tea with the bright flavors of lemon and orange. It's a perfect beverage to cool down and enjoy on hot summer days.

BEETROOT AND BERRY JUICE

Ingredients:

- 1 medium beetroot, peeled and chopped

- 1 cup mixed berries (such as strawberries, blueberries, and raspberries)

- 1 tablespoon lemon juice

- 1-2 tablespoons honey or maple syrup (adjust to taste)

- 1 cup water

- Ice cubes

Instructions:

1. Place the chopped beetroot, mixed berries, lemon juice, honey or maple syrup, and water in a blender.

2. Blend on high speed until the mixture is smooth and well combined.

3. If desired, strain the juice through a fine-mesh sieve to remove any pulp or seeds. This step is optional, and you can skip it if you prefer a thicker juice with more fiber.

4. Taste the juice and adjust the sweetness or tartness by adding more honey, maple syrup, or lemon juice if desired.

5. Fill glasses with ice cubes and pour the Beetroot and Berry Juice into the glasses.

6. Serve the juice chilled and enjoy!

This Beetroot and Berry Juice is a vibrant and nutritious drink that combines the earthy sweetness of beetroot with the natural sweetness of mixed berries. It's packed with antioxidants and vitamins, making it a healthy and refreshing choice for a juice.

Certainly! Here are the recipes for Mango Tango Smoothie with Greek Yogurt and Fresh Orange Juice with Ginger:

MANGO TANGO SMOOTHIE WITH GREEK YOGURT

Ingredients:

- 1 ripe mango, peeled and diced

- 1 ripe banana

- 1/2 cup Greek yogurt

- 1/2 cup orange juice

- 1/2 cup milk (dairy or plant-based)

- 1 tablespoon honey or maple syrup (adjust to taste)

- Ice cubes (optional, for a colder smoothie)

Instructions:

1. Place the diced mango, banana, Greek yogurt, orange juice, milk, and honey or maple syrup in a blender.

2. Blend on high speed until the mixture is smooth and creamy. If desired, add ice cubes and blend again until the smoothie is chilled.

3. Taste the smoothie and adjust the sweetness by adding more honey or maple syrup if desired.

4. Pour the Mango Tango Smoothie with Greek Yogurt into glasses and serve immediately.

This Mango Tango Smoothie with Greek Yogurt is a tropical and creamy treat that combines the sweetness of mangoes with the creaminess of Greek yogurt. The addition of banana, orange juice, and honey or maple syrup creates a well-balanced and delicious smoothie.

FRESH ORANGE JUICE WITH GINGER

Ingredients:

- 4-5 oranges

- 1-inch piece of fresh ginger, peeled and grated

- 1-2 tablespoons honey or maple syrup (adjust to taste)

- Ice cubes

Instructions:

1. Juice the oranges using a citrus juicer or a manual juicer to extract the fresh orange juice.

2. Pour the orange juice into a pitcher or a jar.

3. Add the grated ginger to the orange juice.

4. Stir in honey or maple syrup, adjusting the sweetness to your preference.

5. Stir the orange juice and ginger mixture well to combine the flavors.

6. Place the pitcher or jar in the refrigerator for at least 30 minutes to allow the flavors to meld together.

7. Once chilled, fill glasses with ice cubes and pour the Fresh Orange Juice with Ginger into the glasses.

8. Serve the juice chilled and enjoy!

This Fresh Orange Juice with Ginger is a revitalizing and invigorating drink that combines the natural sweetness of oranges with the warmth and spiciness of ginger. It's a refreshing beverage to enjoy in the morning or throughout the day, providing a burst of flavor and a dose of vitamin C.

BLUEBERRY LAVENDER LEMONADE

Here's a recipe for Blueberry Lavender Lemonade:

Ingredients:

- 1 cup fresh blueberries

- 1/4 cup dried lavender flowers

- 1 cup freshly squeezed lemon juice (about 4-6 lemons)

- 1/2 cup honey or maple syrup (adjust to taste)

- 4 cups water

- Ice cubes

- Fresh blueberries and lavender sprigs for garnish (optional)

Instructions:

1. In a small saucepan, combine the blueberries and dried lavender flowers with 1 cup of water. Bring the mixture to a boil over medium heat.

2. Reduce the heat to low and let the blueberries and lavender simmer for about 10 minutes, or until the blueberries burst and release their juices.

3. Remove the saucepan from heat and strain the blueberry-lavender mixture into a pitcher or a large jar, using a fine-mesh sieve to separate the liquid from the solids. Press the blueberries and lavender flowers with the back of a spoon to extract as much liquid as possible.

4. Add the freshly squeezed lemon juice, honey or maple syrup, and remaining 3 cups of water to the pitcher. Stir well to combine.

5. Taste the lemonade and adjust the sweetness by adding more honey or maple syrup if desired.

6. Place the pitcher in the refrigerator to chill for at least 1-2 hours.

7. Once chilled, fill glasses with ice cubes and pour the Blueberry Lavender Lemonade into the glasses.

8. Garnish each glass with fresh blueberries and a sprig of lavender, if desired.

9. Serve the Blueberry Lavender Lemonade chilled and enjoy!

This Blueberry Lavender Lemonade is a refreshing and aromatic twist on classic lemonade. The combination of sweet blueberries, fragrant lavender, and tangy lemon creates a delightful and visually appealing beverage that is perfect for summer gatherings or any time you want a refreshing drink with a touch of elegance.

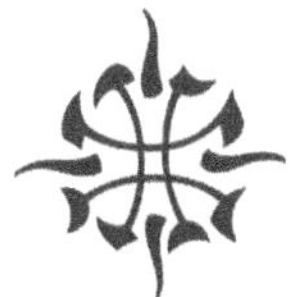

Chapter 8

Easy Weeknight Meals

One-Pan Air-Fried Chicken and Vegetables

Here's a recipe for One-Pan Air-Fried Chicken and Vegetables:

Ingredients:

- 4 boneless, skinless chicken breasts

- 2 cups mixed vegetables (such as broccoli florets, bell peppers, carrots, and zucchini), chopped into bite-sized pieces

- 2 tablespoons olive oil

- 1 teaspoon garlic powder

- 1 teaspoon paprika

- 1/2 teaspoon salt

- 1/4 teaspoon black pepper

- Optional toppings: Fresh herbs (such as parsley or basil), lemon wedges

Instructions:

1. Preheat your air fryer to 400°F (200°C).

2. In a large bowl, combine the olive oil, garlic powder, paprika, salt, and black pepper. Mix well to create a marinade.

3. Add the chicken breasts to the marinade and toss until they are coated evenly. Let the chicken marinate for about 10-15 minutes.

4. Place the marinated chicken breasts in a single layer in the air fryer basket.

5. In the same bowl, add the mixed vegetables and toss them with any remaining marinade.

6. Place the seasoned vegetables around the chicken in the air fryer basket.

7. Cook the chicken and vegetables in the air fryer at 400°F (200°C) for 15-20 minutes, or until the chicken is cooked through and the vegetables are tender. Flip the chicken halfway through cooking to ensure even browning.

8. Once cooked, remove the chicken and vegetables from the air fryer and transfer them to a serving plate.

9. If desired, garnish with fresh herbs and serve with lemon wedges for an extra burst of flavor.

10. Enjoy your delicious One-Pan Air-Fried Chicken and Vegetables!

This recipe allows you to make a complete meal with juicy air-fried chicken breasts and flavorful roasted vegetables—all in one pan. It's a convenient and healthy option that requires minimal cleanup and delivers a satisfying and well-rounded dish.

Here are the recipes for Salmon and Asparagus Foil Packets and Teriyaki Tofu Stir-Fry:

SALMON AND ASPARAGUS FOIL PACKETS

Ingredients:

- 2 salmon fillets

- 1 bunch asparagus, trimmed

- 2 tablespoons olive oil

- 2 cloves garlic, minced

- 1 lemon, sliced

- Salt and pepper, to taste

- Fresh dill or parsley, for garnish

Instructions:

1. Preheat your oven to 400°F (200°C).

2. Cut two large sheets of aluminum foil, enough to wrap each salmon fillet and asparagus.

3. Place one salmon fillet in the center of each sheet of foil. Arrange a handful of trimmed asparagus next to the salmon.

4. Drizzle the salmon and asparagus with olive oil, and sprinkle minced garlic evenly over them. Squeeze the juice of half a lemon over each fillet.

5. Season with salt and pepper to taste.

6. Fold the sides of the foil over the salmon and asparagus, creating a packet. Fold the edges tightly to seal the packet.

7. Place the foil packets on a baking sheet and bake in the preheated oven for about 15-20 minutes, or until the salmon is cooked through and flakes easily with a fork.

8. Carefully open the foil packets, being cautious of the steam, and transfer the salmon and asparagus to plates.

9. Garnish with fresh dill or parsley and serve with lemon slices.

10. Enjoy your delicious Salmon and Asparagus Foil Packets!

This recipe creates a flavorful and healthy meal with tender salmon and perfectly cooked asparagus. The foil packets help seal in the moisture and flavors, resulting in a delicious and fuss-free dish.

TERIYAKI TOFU STIR-FRY

Ingredients:

- 1 block of firm tofu, drained and cubed

- 2 tablespoons soy sauce

- 2 tablespoons teriyaki sauce

- 1 tablespoon sesame oil

- 1 tablespoon vegetable oil

- 1 garlic clove, minced

- 1 teaspoon grated ginger

- 1 bell pepper, sliced

- 1 cup broccoli florets

- 1 carrot, sliced

- 1/2 cup snap peas

- 2 green onions, chopped (optional)

- Sesame seeds, for garnish

Instructions:

1. In a bowl, combine the soy sauce, teriyaki sauce, sesame oil, minced garlic, and grated ginger. Mix well to create the marinade.

2. Add the tofu cubes to the marinade and gently toss to coat. Let the tofu marinate for about 15-30 minutes.

3. Heat the vegetable oil in a large skillet or wok over medium-high heat.

4. Add the marinated tofu to the skillet and cook for about 5 minutes, flipping occasionally, until the tofu is browned and crispy on the outside.

5. Remove the tofu from the skillet and set aside.

6. In the same skillet, add the sliced bell pepper, broccoli florets, carrot slices, and snap peas. Stir-fry the vegetables for about 5-7 minutes, or until they are tender-crisp.

7. Return the tofu to the skillet with the stir-fried vegetables and pour any remaining marinade over the mixture.

8. Stir-fry for another 2-3 minutes, allowing the tofu and vegetables to absorb the flavors of the sauce.

9. Sprinkle chopped green onions and sesame seeds over the stir-fry for added freshness and crunch.

10. Serve the Teriyaki Tofu Stir-Fry over steamed rice or noodles, and enjoy!

This Teriyaki Tofu Stir-Fry is a flavorful and satisfying plant-based dish that combines tender tofu, crisp vegetables, and a delicious teriyaki sauce. It's a versatile recipe that can be customized with your favorite vegetables and enjoyed as a wholesome and tasty meal.

SHRIMP SCAMPI WITH LINGUINE

Ingredients:

- 8 ounces linguine pasta

- 1 pound large shrimp, peeled and deveined

- 4 tablespoons butter

- 4 cloves garlic, minced

- 1/2 cup chicken broth

- 1/4 cup dry white wine (optional)

- 2 tablespoons freshly squeezed lemon juice

- 1/4 teaspoon red pepper flakes (adjust to taste)

- Salt and pepper, to taste

- Fresh parsley, chopped (for garnish)

- Grated Parmesan cheese (optional)

Instructions:

1. Cook the linguine pasta according to the package instructions until al dente. Drain and set aside.

2. In a large skillet, melt the butter over medium heat. Add the minced garlic and sauté for about 1 minute, until fragrant.

3. Add the shrimp to the skillet and cook for 2-3 minutes on each side until they turn pink and opaque. Remove the shrimp from the skillet and set aside.

4. In the same skillet, add the chicken broth, white wine (if using), lemon juice, and red pepper flakes. Season with salt and pepper to taste.

5. Bring the liquid to a simmer and cook for 2-3 minutes to allow the flavors to meld together.

6. Add the cooked linguine to the skillet and toss to coat the pasta with the sauce.

7. Return the cooked shrimp to the skillet and gently toss with the pasta and sauce until everything is well combined.

8. Remove from heat and garnish with freshly chopped parsley and grated Parmesan cheese, if desired.

9. Serve the Shrimp Scampi with Linguine immediately and enjoy!

This classic Italian dish features succulent shrimp in a garlic and butter sauce, served over linguine pasta. It's a delightful combination of flavors and textures that is sure to impress.

BBQ Chicken Quesadillas

Ingredients:

- 2 cups cooked chicken, shredded or diced

- 1/2 cup BBQ sauce

- 4 large flour tortillas

- 2 cups shredded cheddar cheese

- 1/4 cup red onion, thinly sliced

- Fresh cilantro, chopped (for garnish)

- Sour cream and guacamole (optional, for serving)

Instructions:

1. In a bowl, combine the cooked chicken with the BBQ sauce, ensuring all the chicken is coated.

2. Heat a large skillet or griddle over medium heat.

3. Place one tortilla in the skillet and sprinkle half of the shredded cheese evenly over the tortilla.

4. Spoon half of the BBQ chicken mixture onto one half of the tortilla. Top with sliced red onion and a sprinkle of fresh cilantro.

5. Fold the tortilla in half, covering the filling, and press gently.

6. Cook for 2-3 minutes on each side, or until the tortilla is golden brown and the cheese is melted.

7. Remove the quesadilla from the skillet and transfer it to a cutting board. Let it cool for a minute before slicing into wedges.

8. Repeat the process with the remaining tortilla and filling ingredients.

9. Serve the BBQ Chicken Quesadillas with sour cream, guacamole, and additional cilantro if desired.

10. Enjoy the delicious BBQ Chicken Quesadillas as a tasty and satisfying meal or appetizer!

This recipe combines tender BBQ chicken, melted cheese, and tangy red onions in a crispy tortilla. It's a flavorful and easy-to-make dish that is perfect for a quick lunch or dinner.

Thai Basil Chicken Stir-Fry

Ingredients:

- 1 pound boneless, skinless chicken breasts, sliced into thin strips

- 2 tablespoons vegetable oil

- 4 cloves garlic, minced

- 2 Thai bird's eye chilies, thinly sliced (adjust to taste)

- 1 red bell pepper, thinly sliced

- 1 yellow bell pepper, thinly sliced

- 1 onion, thinly sliced

- 1 cup fresh Thai basil leaves

- 3 tablespoons soy sauce

- 1 tablespoon oyster sauce

- 1 tablespoon fish sauce

- 1 teaspoon sugar

- Cooked rice, for serving

Instructions:

1. Heat the vegetable oil in a large skillet or wok over medium-high heat.

2. Add the minced garlic and sliced Thai chilies to the skillet and stir-fry for about 30 seconds, until fragrant.

3. Add the chicken strips to the skillet and cook for 4-5 minutes, or until the chicken is cooked through and no longer pink.

4. Push the chicken to one side of the skillet and add the sliced bell peppers and onion to the other side. Stir-fry the vegetables for about 2-3 minutes until they are slightly tender.

5. In a small bowl, mix together the soy sauce, oyster sauce, fish sauce, and sugar.

6. Pour the sauce mixture over the chicken and vegetables in the skillet. Stir-fry everything together for another minute or two, ensuring the chicken and vegetables are coated in the sauce.

7. Remove the skillet from heat and stir in the fresh Thai basil leaves. The heat from the dish will wilt the basil.

8. Serve the Thai Basil Chicken Stir-Fry over steamed rice and enjoy!

This Thai-inspired stir-fry features tender chicken, colorful bell peppers, and aromatic Thai basil leaves. It's a flavorful and aromatic dish that pairs well with steamed rice for a complete meal.

Enjoy preparing and savoring these delicious recipes!

Certainly! Here are the recipes for Margherita Panini and Pork Chops with Apple Compote:

MARGHERITA PANINI

Ingredients:

- 4 ciabatta rolls or other bread of your choice

- 1/4 cup basil pesto

- 2 large tomatoes, sliced

- 8 ounces fresh mozzarella cheese, sliced

- Fresh basil leaves

- Olive oil, for brushing

Instructions:

1. Preheat a panini press or grill pan.

2. Slice the ciabatta rolls in half horizontally to create a top and bottom piece for each panini.

3. Spread a thin layer of basil pesto on the cut side of each roll.

4. On the bottom half of each roll, layer tomato slices, fresh mozzarella slices, and a few basil leaves.

5. Place the top half of the roll on the ingredients to form a sandwich.

6. Brush the outside of each panini with olive oil.

7. Place the panini on the preheated panini press or grill pan and cook for about 3-4 minutes, or until the bread is toasted and the cheese has melted.

8. Remove the panini from the press or pan and let them cool for a minute or two.

9. Slice the panini in half and serve them warm.

10. Enjoy the delicious Margherita Panini as a flavorful and satisfying meal!

This panini features the classic Margherita pizza flavors, with fresh tomatoes, mozzarella cheese, and basil pesto. Grilling the panini gives it a crispy exterior and a melty, gooey interior.

PORK CHOPS WITH APPLE COMPOTE

Ingredients:

- 4 boneless pork chops

- Salt and pepper, to taste

- 2 tablespoons butter

- 2 apples, peeled, cored, and sliced

- 2 tablespoons brown sugar

- 1/2 teaspoon cinnamon

- 1/4 cup apple cider or apple juice

- 1 tablespoon lemon juice

Instructions:

1. Season the pork chops with salt and pepper on both sides.

2. In a large skillet, melt the butter over medium-high heat.

3. Add the pork chops to the skillet and cook for about 4-5 minutes on each side, or until they reach an internal temperature of 145°F (63°C). Adjust the cooking time depending on the thickness of the pork chops.

4. Remove the pork chops from the skillet and set them aside to rest.

5. In the same skillet, add the sliced apples, brown sugar, cinnamon, apple cider or apple juice, and lemon juice.

6. Cook the apple mixture over medium heat for about 5-7 minutes, or until the apples are tender and the liquid has thickened slightly.

7. Stir the apple compote occasionally to ensure it cooks evenly.

8. Once the apple compote is ready, remove it from the heat.

9. Serve the pork chops topped with the warm apple compote.

10. Enjoy the Pork Chops with Apple Compote as a delicious and comforting meal!

This recipe pairs tender and juicy pork chops with a sweet and tangy apple compote. The combination of flavors creates a delightful contrast that is sure to please your taste buds.

Enjoy preparing and savoring these delicious recipes!

Certainly! Here are the recipes for Spaghetti Aglio e Olio and Black Bean and Corn Stuffed Sweet Potatoes:

SPAGHETTI AGLIO E OLIO

Ingredients:

- 8 ounces spaghetti

- 1/4 cup olive oil

- 6 cloves garlic, thinly sliced

- 1/2 teaspoon red pepper flakes (adjust to taste)

- Salt, to taste

- Fresh parsley, chopped (for garnish)

- Grated Parmesan cheese (optional)

Instructions:

1. Cook the spaghetti according to the package instructions until al dente. Drain and set aside.

2. In a large skillet, heat the olive oil over medium heat.

3. Add the sliced garlic and red pepper flakes to the skillet. Cook for about 2-3 minutes, stirring frequently, until the

garlic is golden brown and fragrant. Be careful not to burn the garlic.

4. Add the cooked spaghetti to the skillet and toss to coat the pasta with the garlic-infused oil.

5. Season with salt to taste and toss again to distribute the flavors evenly.

6. Remove the skillet from heat and garnish the spaghetti aglio e olio with freshly chopped parsley.

7. Serve the spaghetti aglio e olio immediately. You can sprinkle some grated Parmesan cheese on top, if desired.

8. Enjoy the simple and flavorful Spaghetti Aglio e Olio!

This classic Italian dish features spaghetti tossed in a garlic-infused olive oil, with a hint of red pepper flakes for a touch of heat. It's a quick and easy recipe that highlights the simplicity of quality ingredients.

BLACK BEAN AND CORN STUFFED SWEET POTATOES

Ingredients:

- 4 medium sweet potatoes

- 1 tablespoon olive oil

- 1 small onion, diced

- 2 cloves garlic, minced

- 1 bell pepper, diced

- 1 cup canned black beans, rinsed and drained

- 1 cup frozen corn kernels, thawed

- 1 teaspoon cumin

- 1/2 teaspoon chili powder (adjust to taste)

- Salt and pepper, to taste

- Fresh cilantro, chopped (for garnish)

- Lime wedges, for serving

Instructions:

1. Preheat the oven to 400°F (200°C).

2. Place the sweet potatoes on a baking sheet and prick them with a fork. Bake for about 45-60 minutes, or until the sweet potatoes are tender when pierced with a fork.

3. While the sweet potatoes are baking, prepare the black bean and corn filling.

4. In a large skillet, heat the olive oil over medium heat.

5. Add the diced onion, minced garlic, and diced bell pepper to the skillet. Sauté for about 5 minutes, or until the vegetables are softened.

6. Add the black beans, corn kernels, cumin, chili powder, salt, and pepper to the skillet. Stir well to combine.

7. Cook the filling for another 5 minutes, stirring occasionally, until the flavors meld together. Adjust the seasoning to taste.

8. Once the sweet potatoes are cooked, remove them from the oven and let them cool slightly.

9. Slice each sweet potato lengthwise and gently mash the flesh with a fork.

10. Spoon the black bean and corn filling into the sweet potato halves, dividing it evenly among them.

11. Garnish with fresh chopped cilantro.

12. Serve the Black Bean and Corn Stuffed Sweet Potatoes with lime wedges on the side for squeezing over the top.

13. Enjoy the flavorful and nutritious Black Bean and Corn Stuffed Sweet Potatoes as a tasty and satisfying meal!

This recipe combines the sweetness of roasted sweet potatoes with a flavorful and hearty black bean and corn filling. It's a delicious and nutritious dish that can be enjoyed as a main course or a side dish.

Enjoy preparing and savoring these delicious recipes!

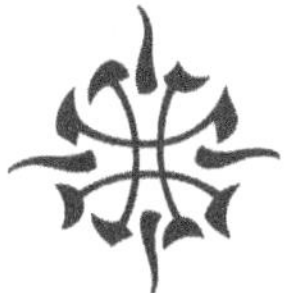

Chapter 9

Meal Planning and Tips for Seniors

GLOSSARY OF INGREDIENTS

1. Plan Ahead: Take some time to plan your meals for the week. This will help you stay organized and ensure you have all the necessary ingredients on hand.

2. Balance Nutrients: Aim for a balanced diet that includes a variety of nutrients. Include fruits, vegetables, whole grains, lean proteins, and healthy fats in your meals.

3. Portion Control: Be mindful of portion sizes to avoid overeating. Use smaller plates and bowls to help control portion sizes.

4. Include Protein: Protein is essential for maintaining muscle mass and overall health. Include protein-rich foods such as lean meats, poultry, fish, eggs, beans, and tofu in your meals.

5. Include Fiber: Fiber aids in digestion and helps maintain bowel regularity. Include high-fiber foods like whole grains, fruits, vegetables, and legumes in your meals.

6. Stay Hydrated: Drink plenty of water throughout the day to stay hydrated. Limit sugary drinks and opt for water, herbal tea, or low-sodium broth.

7. Cook in Batches: Consider cooking larger portions and storing leftovers in individual containers for future meals. This can save time and ensure you have nutritious meals readily available.

8. Use Convenience Foods Wisely: While convenience foods can be helpful, choose healthier options with minimal added sugars, sodium, and unhealthy fats. Look for pre-cut fruits and vegetables or frozen options without added sauces.

9. Seek Social Connections: Eating meals with others can enhance the dining experience. Consider joining community meal programs or organizing regular meals with friends or family.

Glossary of Ingredients

Here are some common ingredients you may come across in recipes:

1. All-Purpose Flour: A versatile flour used in baking and cooking.

2. Baking Powder: A leavening agent used in baking to help dough or batter rise.

3. Olive Oil: A healthy fat used for cooking and dressing salads.

4. Garlic: A pungent bulb used as a flavoring agent in many dishes.

5. Onion: A vegetable used as a flavor base in various cuisines.

6. Bell Pepper: A colorful, sweet vegetable used in salads, stir-fries, and other dishes.

7. Cumin: A spice with a warm, earthy flavor commonly used in Mexican, Indian, and Middle Eastern cuisines.

8. Basil: A fragrant herb with a sweet and slightly peppery flavor used in Italian and Mediterranean cuisines.

9. Parmesan Cheese: A hard, aged cheese with a nutty flavor often used as a topping or in sauces.

10. Quinoa: A nutritious grain-like seed that can be used as a substitute for rice or added to salads and soups.

11. Salmon: A fatty fish rich in omega-3 fatty acids and protein, commonly baked, grilled, or pan-seared.

12. Kale: A dark, leafy green vegetable packed with nutrients and often used in salads, stir-fries, and smoothies.

This glossary includes just a few ingredients, but there are countless others used in various cuisines. Exploring new ingredients can add excitement and variety to your meals.

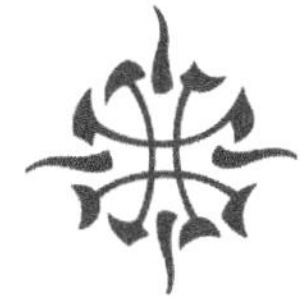

Chapter 10

Conclusion

In conclusion, meal planning and preparation for seniors can be a rewarding and enjoyable process. By following these meal planning tips and incorporating a variety of nutritious ingredients into your recipes, you can maintain a healthy and balanced diet. Planning ahead, balancing nutrients, controlling portion sizes, and including protein and fiber are all important considerations. Additionally, staying hydrated, cooking in batches, using convenience foods wisely, and seeking social connections during meals can further enhance your overall dining experience. With a glossary of common ingredients, you can expand your culinary knowledge and experiment with new flavors. Remember, mealtime is not only about nourishing your body but also about savoring delicious and wholesome meals. Enjoy the process of planning, preparing, and sharing meals with loved ones as you prioritize your well-being and enjoyment of food.